Osteogenesis and Bone Regeneration

Edited by Haisheng Yang

Published in London, United Kingdom

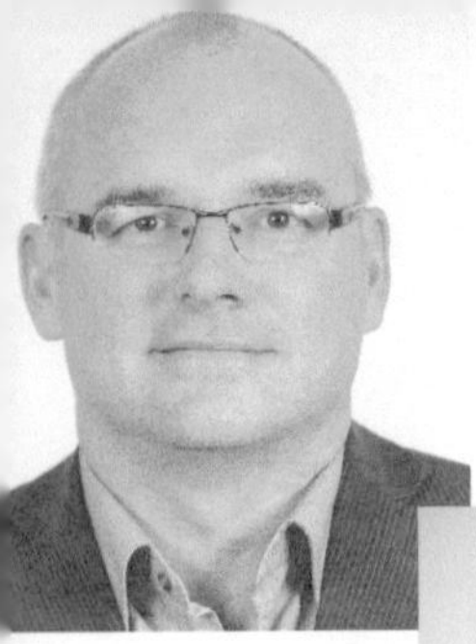
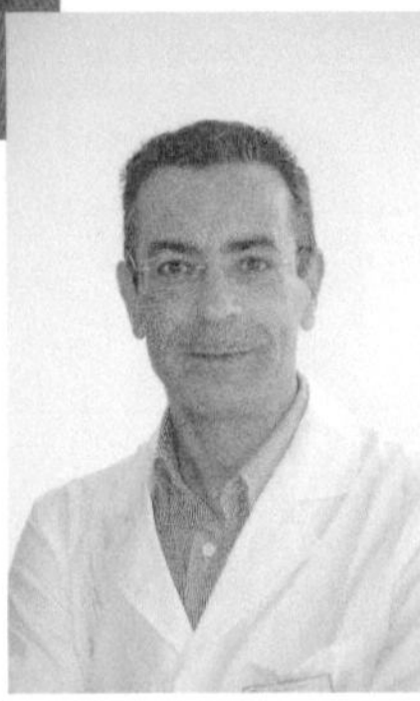
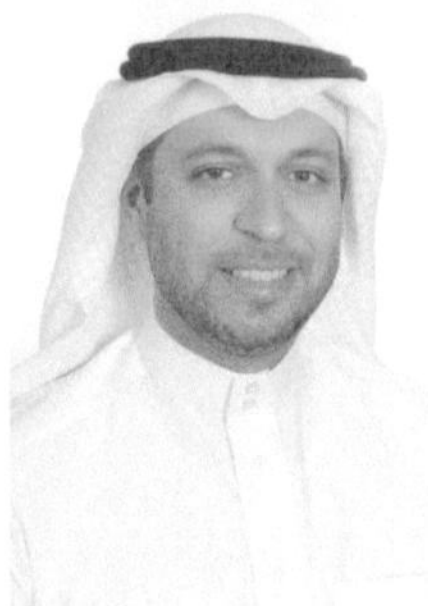
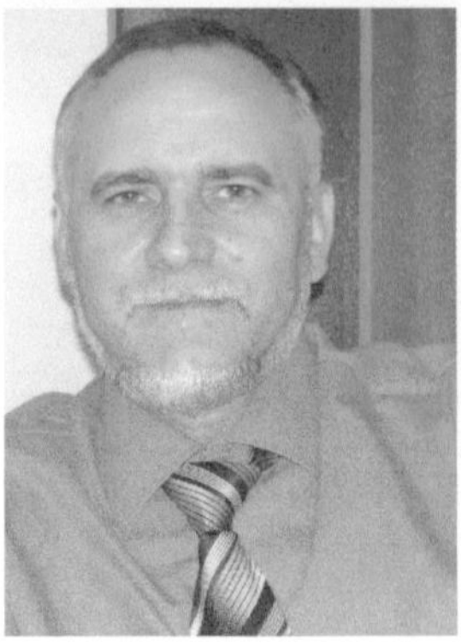
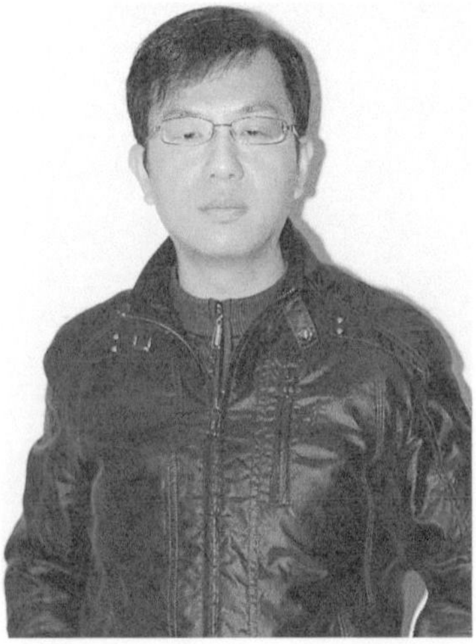
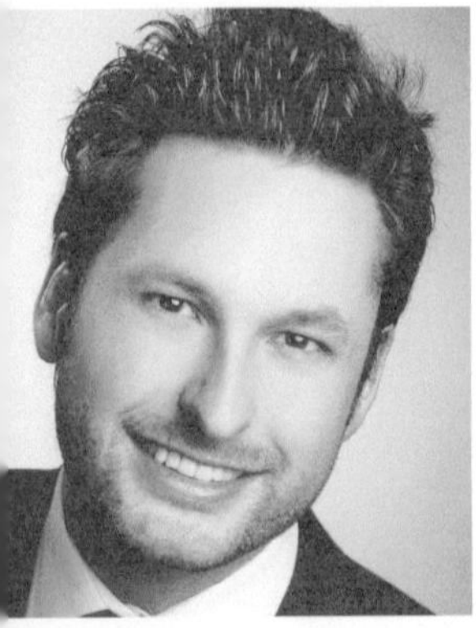
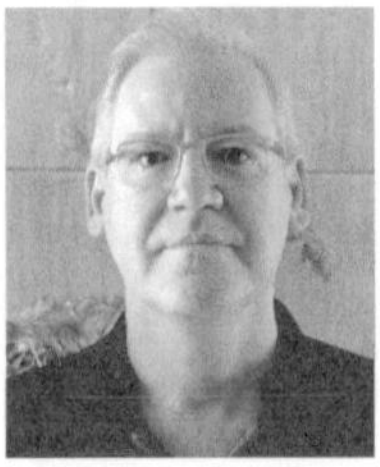

IntechOpen

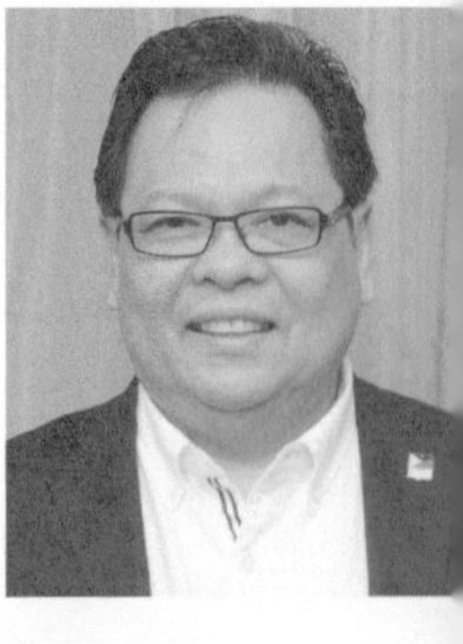
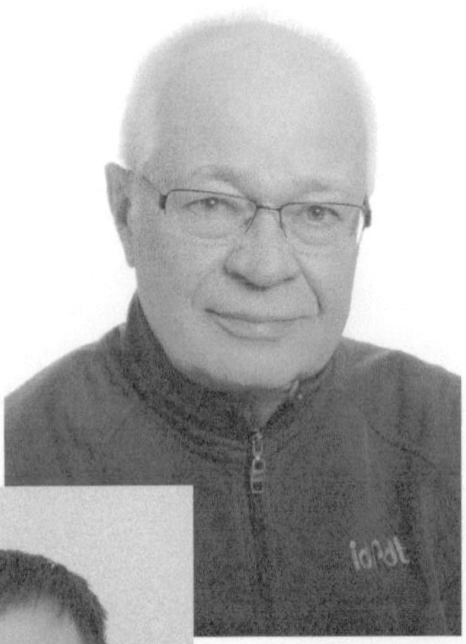
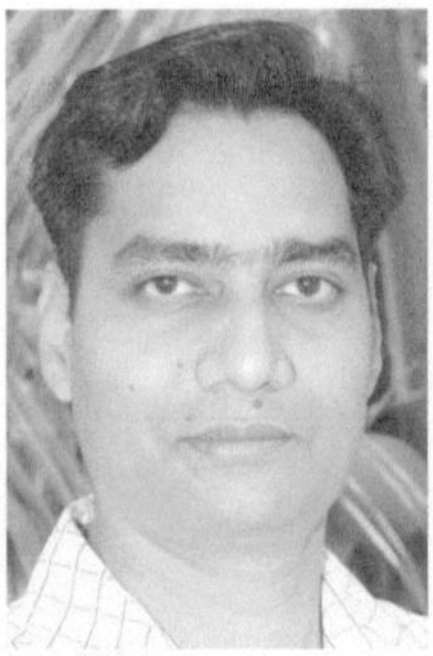
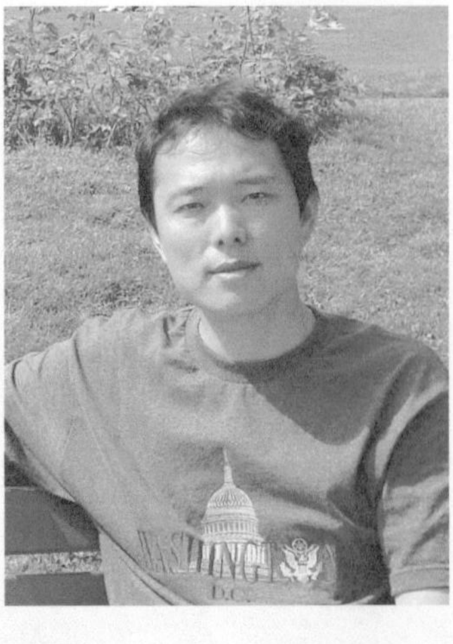
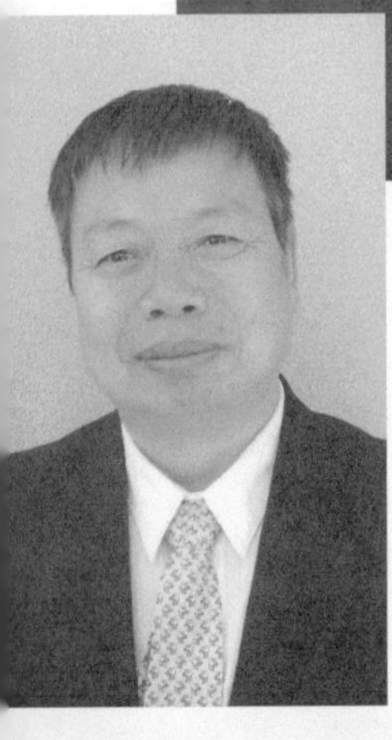
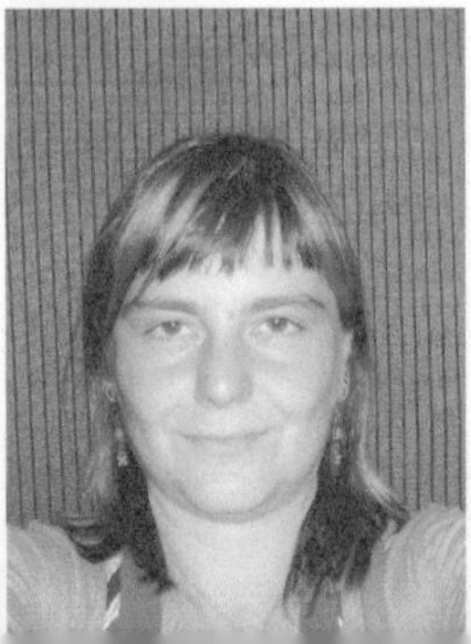

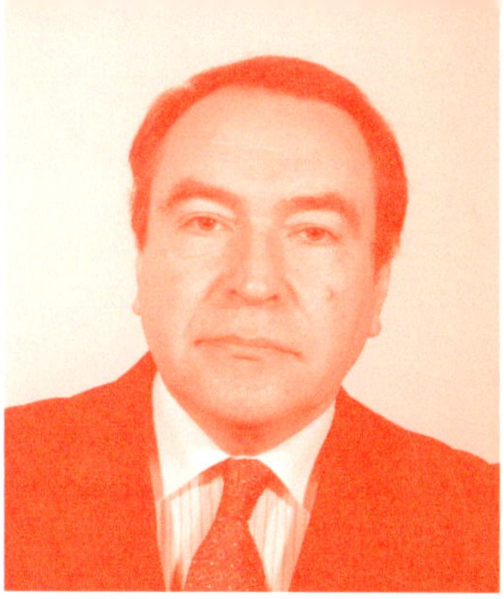
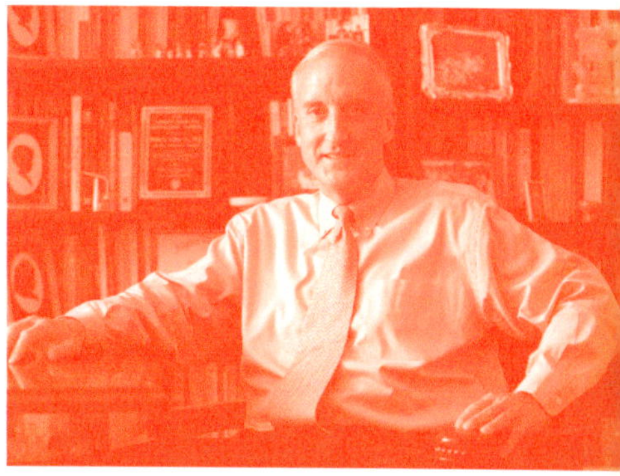
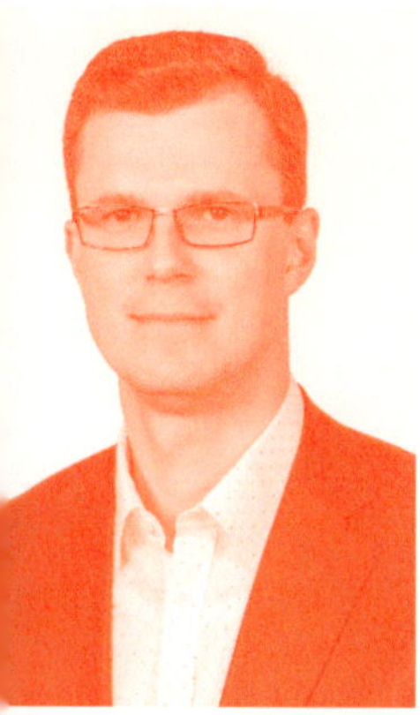
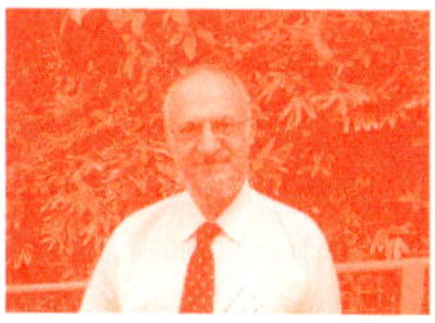
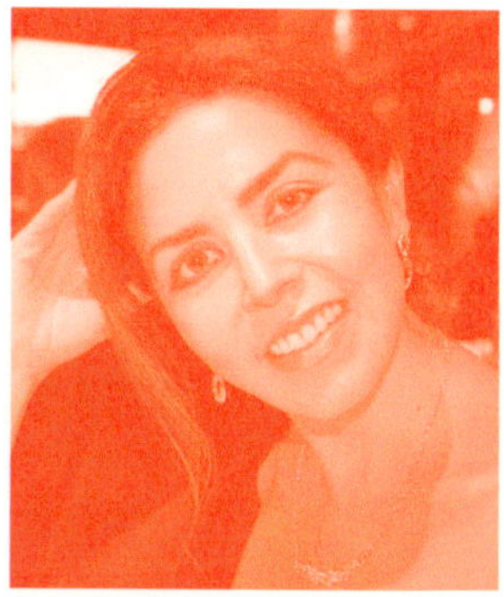

Supporting open minds since 2005

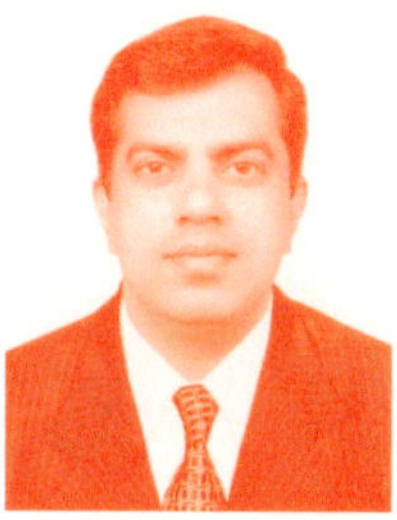
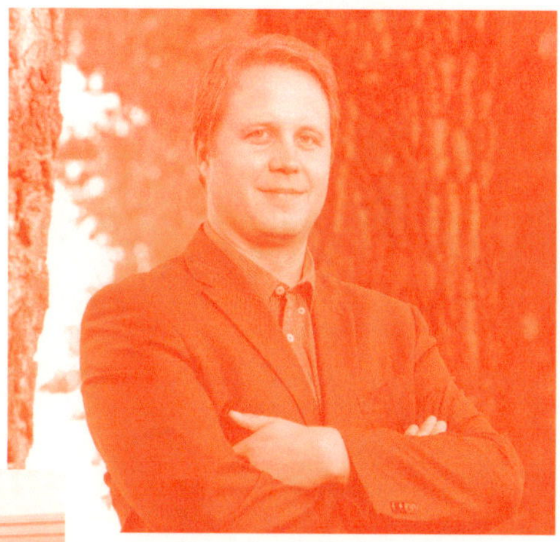
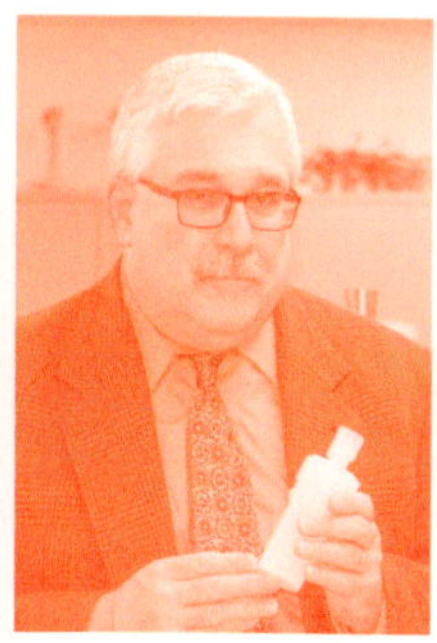
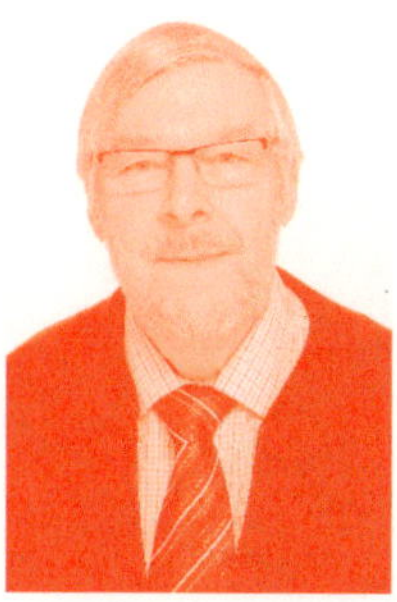
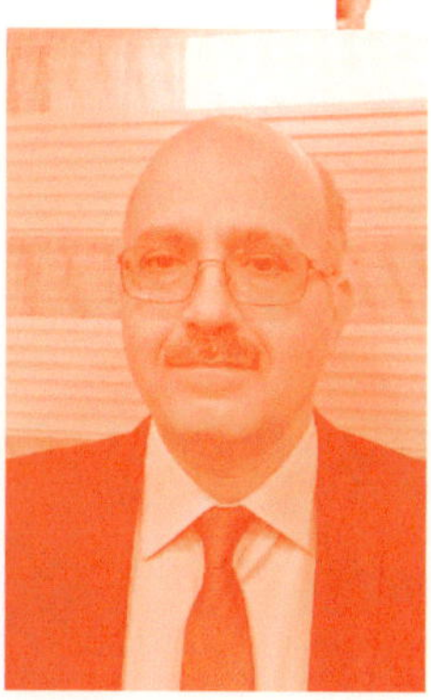
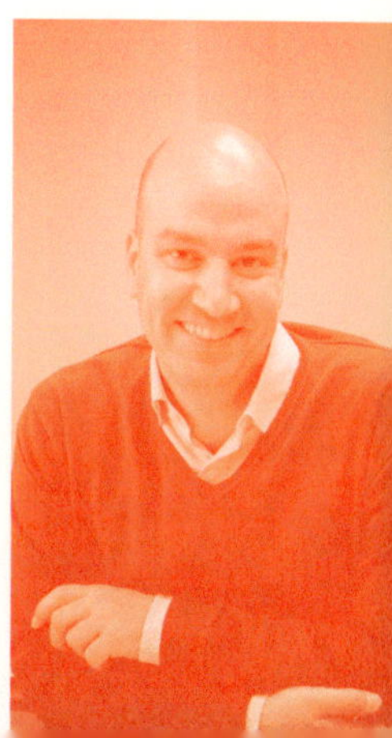
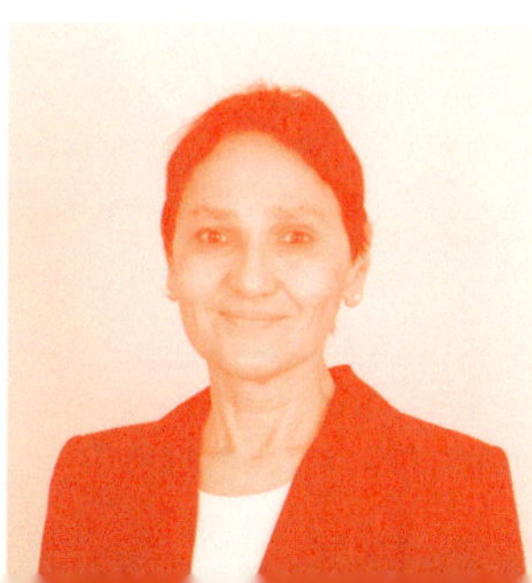

Osteogenesis and Bone Regeneration
http://dx.doi.org/10.5772/intechopen.73955
Edited by Haisheng Yang

Contributors
Yandong Mu, Chenglong Li, Lu Yang, Wei Qing, Yanqin Lu, Jinxiang Han, Firdaus Hariri, Siok Yoong Chin, Jonathan Rengarajoo, Qi Chao Foo, Siti Nur Nabihah Zainul Abidin, Ahmad Fadhli Ahmad Badruddin, Lixin Kan, Yang Jiazhao, Wanbo Zhu, Jinsen Lu, Kai Xie, Shiyuan Shiyuan, Daniela Bueno, Carla Cristina Gomes Pinheiro, Yanqiu Liu, Rosy Setiawati, Paulus Rahardjo

First published in London, United Kingdom, 2019 by IntechOpen
IntechOpen is the global imprint of INTECHOPEN LIMITED, registered in England and Wales, registration number: 11086078, The Shard, 25th floor, 32 London Bridge Street
London, SE19SG – United Kingdom
Printed in Croatia

British Library Cataloguing-in-Publication Data
A catalogue record for this book is available from the British Library

Additional hard copies can be obtained from orders@intechopen.com

Osteogenesis and Bone Regeneration
Edited by Haisheng Yang
p. cm.
Print ISBN 978-1-78985-767-2
Online ISBN 978-1-78985-768-9

For EU product safety concerns:
IN TECH d.o.o., Prolaz Marije Krucifikse Kozulić 3, 51000 Rijeka, Croatia, info@intechopen.com or visit our website at intechopen.com.

Meet the editor

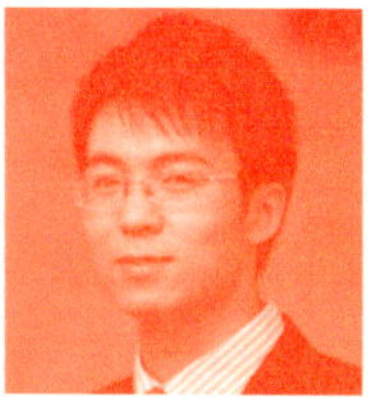

Haisheng Yang, Ph.D., is the Director and BJUT Professor of the Department of Biomedical Engineering, College of Life Science and Bioengineering, Beijing University of Technology. He received his Ph.D. degree in Mechanics/Biomechanics from Harbin Institute of Technology (jointly with University of California, Berkeley). Afterwards, he worked as a Postdoctoral Research Associate in the Purdue Musculoskeletal Biology and Mechanics Lab at the Department of Basic Medical Sciences, Purdue University, USA. He conducted research in the Research Centre of Shriners Hospitals for Children-Canada at McGill University, Canada. Dr. Yang has over 10 years of research experience in orthopedic biomechanics and mechanobiology of bone adaptation and regeneration. He earned an award from Beijing Overseas Talents Aggregation program and is honored as one of the Beijing Specially Recruited Experts.

Contents

Preface

Osteogenesis, the formation of bone or the development of bones, has two major modes — intramembranous ossification and endochondral ossification — and both involve the transformation of a pre-existing mesenchymal tissue into bone tissue. Osteogenesis is a core component of the skeletal system and depends on the well-coordinated proliferation and differentiation of osteogenic cells, including chondrocytes and osteoblasts. Multiple signaling pathways and transcriptional factors tightly regulate the process of osteogenesis. Any abnormities in bone formation could cause severe disorders such as osteogenesis imperfecta (OI) and osteoporosis. Understanding the mechanisms of osteogenesis can be helpful for clinical treatment of all conditions that affect bone formation, from congenital deformities to bone fractures. This book provides the reader with a comprehensive overview of the current developments in osteogenesis, including its underlying biological and mechanobiological mechanisms, its related clinical diseases and treatment strategies, and particularly advanced applications in bone regeneration and tissue engineering.

Funding from the National Natural Science Foundation of China (11702008), Beijing Excellent Talents Funds (2017000020124G277), and Support Plan for High-level Faculties in Beijing Municipal Universities (CIT&TCD201804011) is greatly acknowledged.

Haisheng Yang
Department of Biomedical Engineering,
College of Life Science and Bioengineering,
Intelligent Physiological Measurement and Clinical Translation,
Beijing International Base for Scientific and Technological Cooperation,
Beijing University of Technology, China

Chapter 1

Bone Development and Growth

Rosy Setiawati and Paulus Rahardjo

Abstract

The process of bone formation is called osteogenesis or ossification. After progenitor cells form osteoblastic lines, they proceed with three stages of development of cell differentiation, called proliferation, maturation of matrix, and mineralization. Based on its embryological origin, there are two types of ossification, called intramembranous ossification that occurs in mesenchymal cells that differentiate into osteoblast in the ossification center directly without prior cartilage formation and endochondral ossification in which bone tissue mineralization is formed through cartilage formation first. In intramembranous ossification, bone development occurs directly. In this process, mesenchymal cells proliferate into areas that have high vascularization in embryonic connective tissue in the formation of cell condensation or primary ossification centers. This cell will synthesize bone matrix in the periphery and the mesenchymal cells continue to differentiate into osteoblasts. After that, the bone will be reshaped and replaced by mature lamellar bone. Endochondral ossification will form the center of primary ossification, and the cartilage extends by proliferation of chondrocytes and deposition of cartilage matrix. After this formation, chondrocytes in the central region of the cartilage start to proceed with maturation into hypertrophic chondrocytes. After the primary ossification center is formed, the marrow cavity begins to expand toward the epiphysis. Then the subsequent stages of endochondral ossification will take place in several zones of the bone.

Keywords: osteogenesis, ossification, bone formation, intramembranous ossification, endochondral ossification

1. Introduction

Bone is living tissue that is the hardest among other connective tissues in the body, consists of 50% water. The solid part remainder consisting of various minerals, especially 76% of calcium salt and 33% of cellular material. Bone has vascular tissue and cellular activity products, especially during growth which is very dependent on the blood supply as basic source and hormones that greatly regulate this growth process. Bone-forming cells, osteoblasts, osteoclast play an important role in determining bone growth, thickness of the cortical layer and structural arrangement of the lamellae.

Bone continues to change its internal structure to reach the functional needs and these changes occur through the activity of osteoclasts and osteoblasts. The bone seen from its development can be divided into two processes: first is the intramembranous ossification in which bones form directly in the form of primitive mesenchymal connective tissue, such as the mandible, maxilla and skull bones. Second is the endochondral ossification in which bone tissue replaces a preexisting hyaline cartilage, for example during skull base formation. The same formative cells form two types of bone formation and the final structure is not much different.

Bone growth depends on genetic and environmental factors, including hormonal effects, diet and mechanical factors. The growth rate is not always the same in all parts, for example, faster in the proximal end than the distal humerus because the internal pattern of the spongiosum depends on the direction of bone pressure. The direction of bone formation in the epiphysis plane is determined by the direction and distribution of the pressure line. Increased thickness or width of the bone is caused by deposition of new bone in the form of circumferential lamellae under the periosteum. If bone growth continues, the lamella will be embedded behind the new bone surface and be replaced by the haversian canal system.

2. Bone cells and matrix

Bone is a tissue in which the extracellular matrix has been hardened to accommodate a supporting function. The fundamental components of bone, like all connective tissues, are cells and matrix. Although bone cells compose a small amount of the bone volume, they are crucial to the function of bones. Four types of cells are found within bone tissue: osteoblasts, osteocytes, osteogenic cells, and osteoclasts. They each unique functions and are derived from two different cell lines (**Figure 1** and **Table 1**) [1–7].

- Osteoblast synthesizes the bone matrix and are responsible for its mineralization. They are derived from osteoprogenitor cells, a mesenchymal stem cell line.

- Osteocytes are inactive osteoblasts that have become trapped within the bone they have formed.

- Osteoclasts break down bone matrix through phagocytosis. Predictably, they ruffled border, and the space between the osteoblast and the bone is known as Howship's lacuna.

The balance between osteoblast and osteoclast activity governs bone turnover and ensures that bone is neither overproduced nor overdegraded. These cells build up and break down bone matrix, which is composed of:

- Osteoid, which is the unmineralized matrix composed of type I collagen and gylcosaminoglycans (GAGs).

- Calcium hydroxyapatite, a calcium salt crystal that give bone its strength and rigidity.

Bone is divided into two types that are different structurally and functionally. Most bones of the body consist of both types of bone tissue (**Figure 2**) [1, 2, 8, 9]:

- Compact bone, or cortical bone, mainly serves a mechanical function. This is the area of bone to which ligaments and tendons attach. It is thick and dense.

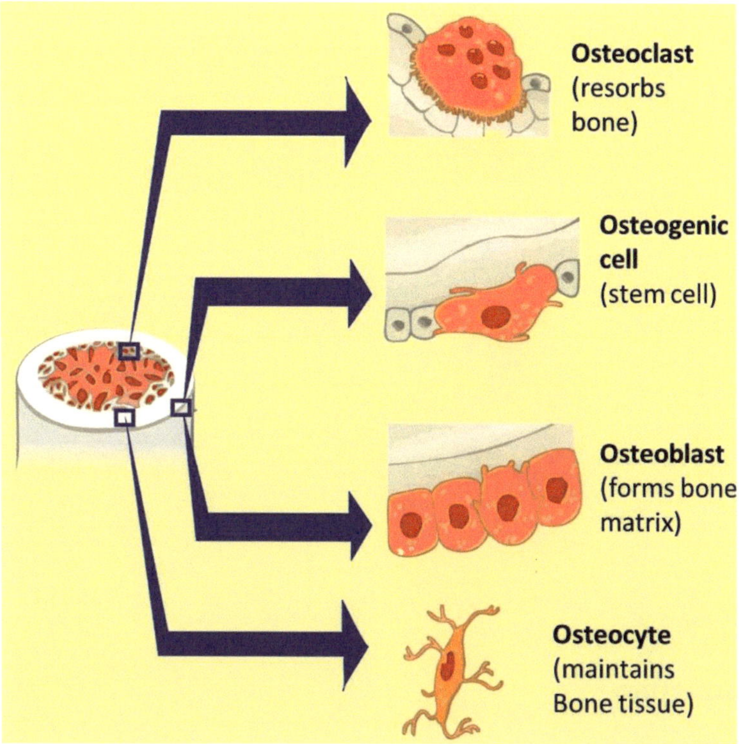

Figure 1.
Development of bone precursor cells. Bone precursor cells are divided into developmental stages, which are 1. mesenchymal stem cell, 2. pre-osteoblast, 3. osteoblast, and 4. mature osteocytes, and 5. osteoclast.

Cell type	Function	Location
Osteogenic cells	Develop in osteoblast	Deep layers of the periosteum and the marrow
Osteoblast	Bone formation	Growing portions of bone, including periosteum and endosteum
Osteocytes	Maintain mineral concentration of matrix	Entrapped in matrix
Osteoclasts	Bone resoprtion	Bone surfaces and at sites of old, injured, or unneeded bone

Table 1.
Bone cells, their function, and locations [1–7].

- Trabecular bone, also known as cancellous bone or spongy bone, mainly serves a metabolic function. This type of bone is located between layers of compact bone and is thin porous. Location within the trabeculae is the bone marrow.

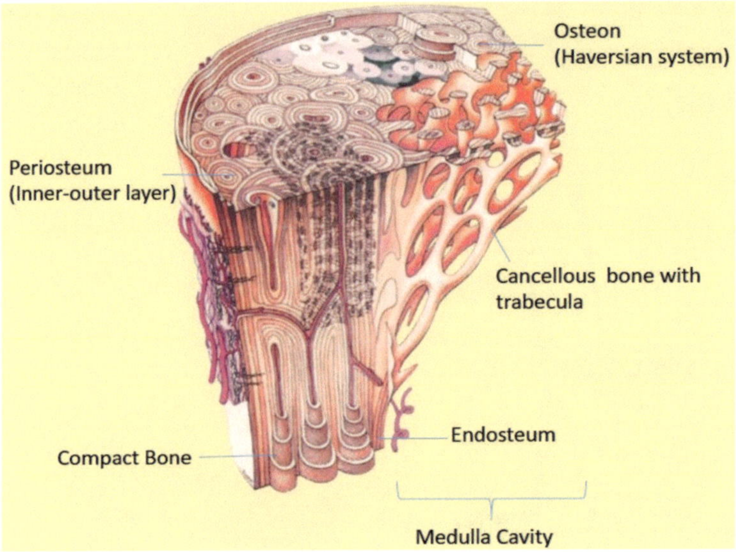

Figure 2.
Structure of a long bone.

3. Bone structure

3.1 Macroscopic bone structure

Long bones are composed of both cortical and cancellous bone tissue. They consist of several areas (**Figure 3**) [3, 4]:

- The epiphysis is located at the end of the long bone and is the parts of the bone that participate in joint surfaces.
- The diaphysis is the shaft of the bone and has walls of cortical bone and an underlying network of trabecular bone.
- The epiphyseal growth plate lies at the interface between the shaft and the epiphysis and is the region in which cartilage proliferates to cause the elongation of the bone.
- The metaphysis is the area in which the shaft of the bone joins the epiphyseal growth plate.

Different areas of the bone are covered by different tissue [4]:

- The epiphysis is lined by a layer of articular cartilage, a specialized form of hyaline cartilage, which serves as protection against friction in the joints.
- The outside of the diaphysis is lined by periosteum, a fibrous external layer onto which muscles, ligaments, and tendons attach.
- The inside of the diaphysis, at the border between the cortical and cancellous bone and lining the trabeculae, is lined by endosteum.

DOI: http://dx.doi.org/10.5772/intechopen.82452

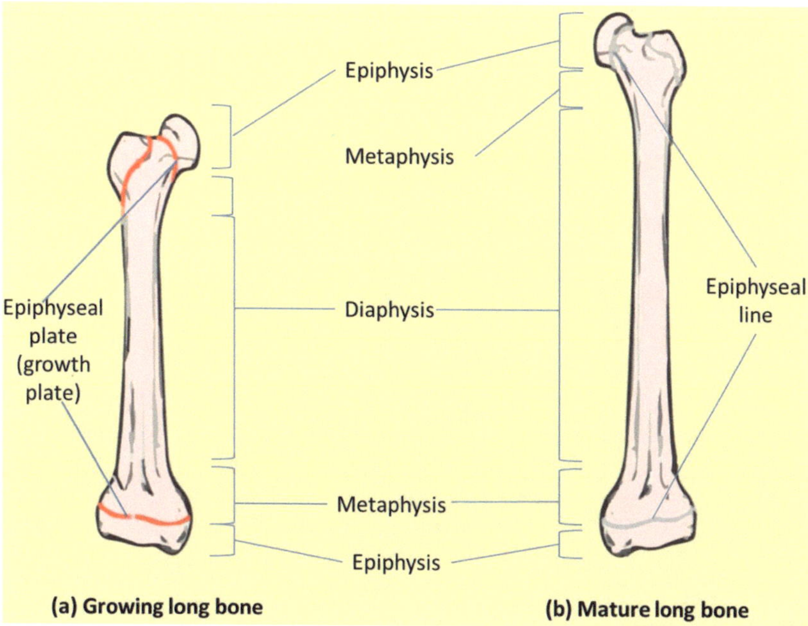

Figure 3.
Bone macrostructure. (a) Growing long bone showing epiphyses, epiphyseal plates, metaphysis and diaphysis. (b) Mature long bone showing epiphyseal lines.

3.2 Microscopic bone structure

Compact bone is organized as parallel columns, known as Haversian systems, which run lengthwise down the axis of long bones. These columns are composed of lamellae, concentric rings of bone, surrounding a central channel, or Haversian canal, that contains the nerves, blood vessels, and lymphatic system of the bone. The parallel Haversian canals are connected to one another by the perpendicular Volkmann's canals.

The lamellae of the Haversian systems are created by osteoblasts. As these cells secrete matrix, they become trapped in spaces called lacunae and become known as osteocytes. Osteocytes communicate with the Haversian canal through cytoplasmic extensions that run through canaliculi, small interconnecting canals (**Figure 4**) [1, 2, 8, 9]:

The layers of a long bone, beginning at the external surface, are therefore:

- Periosteal surface of compact bone
- Outer circumferential lamellae
- Compact bone (Haversian systems)
- Inner circumferential lamellae
- Endosteal surface of compact bone
- Trabecular bone

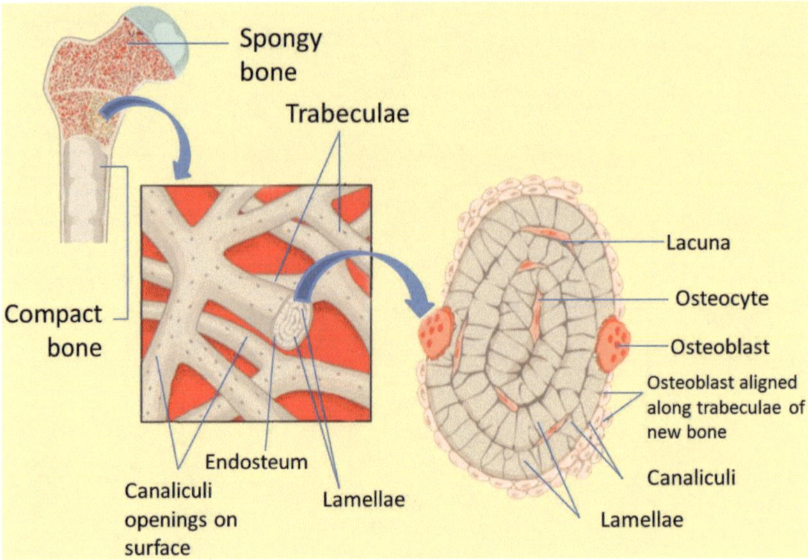

Figure 4.
Bone microstructure. Compact and spongy bone structures.

4. Bone formation

Bone development begins with the replacement of collagenous mesenchymal tissue by bone. This results in the formation of woven bone, a primitive form of bone with randomly organized collagen fibers that is further remodeled into mature lamellar bone, which possesses regular parallel rings of collagen. Lamellar bone is then constantly remodeled by osteoclasts and osteoblasts. Based on the development of bone formation can be divided into two parts, called endochondral and intramembranous bone formation/ossification [1–3, 8].

4.1 Intramembranous bone formation

During intramembranous bone formation, the connective tissue membrane of undifferentiated mesenchymal cells changes into bone and matrix bone cells [10]. In the craniofacial cartilage bones, intramembranous ossification originates from nerve crest cells. The earliest evidence of intramembranous bone formation of the skull occurs in the mandible during the sixth prenatal week. In the eighth week, reinforcement center appears in the calvarial and facial areas in areas where there is a mild stress strength [11].

Intramembranous bone formation is found in the growth of the skull and is also found in the sphenoid and mandible even though it consists of endochondral elements, where the endochondral and intramembranous growth process occurs in the same bone. The basis for either bone formation or bone resorption is the same, regardless of the type of membrane involved.

Sometimes according to where the formation of bone tissue is classified as "periosteal" or "endosteal". Periosteal bone always originates from intramembranous, but endosteal bone can originate from intramembranous as well as endochondral ossification, depending on the location and the way it is formed [3, 12].

4.1.1 The stage of intramembranous bone formation

The statement below is the stage of intramembrane bone formation (**Figure 5**) [3, 4, 11, 12]:

1. An ossification center appears in the fibrous connective tissue membrane. Mesenchymal cells in the embryonic skeleton gather together and begin to differentiate into specialized cells. Some of these cells differentiate into capillaries, while others will become osteogenic cells and osteoblasts, then forming an ossification center.

2. Bone matrix (osteoid) is secreted within the fibrous membrane. Osteoblasts produce osteoid tissue, by means of differentiating osteoblasts from the ectomesenchyme condensation center and producing bone fibrous matrix (osteoid). Then osteoid is mineralized within a few days and trapped osteoblast become osteocytes.

3. Woven bone and periosteum form. The encapsulation of cells and blood vessels occur. When osteoid deposition by osteoblasts continues, the encased cells develop into osteocytes. Accumulating osteoid is laid down between embryonic blood vessels, which form a random network (instead of lamellae) of trabecular. Vascularized mesenchyme condenses on external face of the woven bone and becomes the periosteum.

4. Production of osteoid tissue by membrane cells: osteocytes lose their ability to contribute directly to an increase in bone size, but osteoblasts on the periosteum surface produce more osteoid tissue that thickens the tissue layer on the existing bone surface (for example, appositional bone growth). Formation of a woven bone collar that is later replaced by mature lamellar bone. Spongy bone (diploe), consisting of distinct trabeculae, persists internally and its vascular tissue becomes red marrow.

5. Osteoid calcification: The occurrence of bone matrix mineralization makes bones relatively impermeable to nutrients and metabolic waste. Trapped blood vessels function to supply nutrients to osteocytes as well as bone tissue and eliminate waste products.

6. The formation of an essential membrane of bone which includes a membrane outside the bone called the bone endosteum. Bone endosteum is very important for bone survival. Disruption of the membrane or its vascular tissue can cause bone cell death and bone loss. Bones are very sensitive to pressure. The calcified bones are hard and relatively inflexible.

The matrix or intercellular substance of the bone becomes calcified and becomes a bone in the end. Bone tissue that is found in the periosteum, endosteum, suture, and periodontal membrane (ligaments) is an example of intramembranous bone formation [3, 13].

Intramembranous bone formation occurs in two types of bone: bundle bone and lamellar bone. The bone bundle develops directly in connective tissue that has not been calcified. Osteoblasts, which are differentiated from the mesenchyme, secrete an intercellular substance containing collagen fibrils. This osteoid matrix calcifies by precipitating apatite crystals. Primary ossification centers only show minimal bone calcification density. The apatite crystal deposits are mostly irregular and structured like nets that are contained in the medullary and cortical regions. Mineralization occurs very quickly (several tens of thousands of millimeters per day) and can occur simultaneously in large areas. These apatite deposits increase with time. Bone tissue is only considered mature when the crystalized area is arranged in the same direction as collagen fibrils.

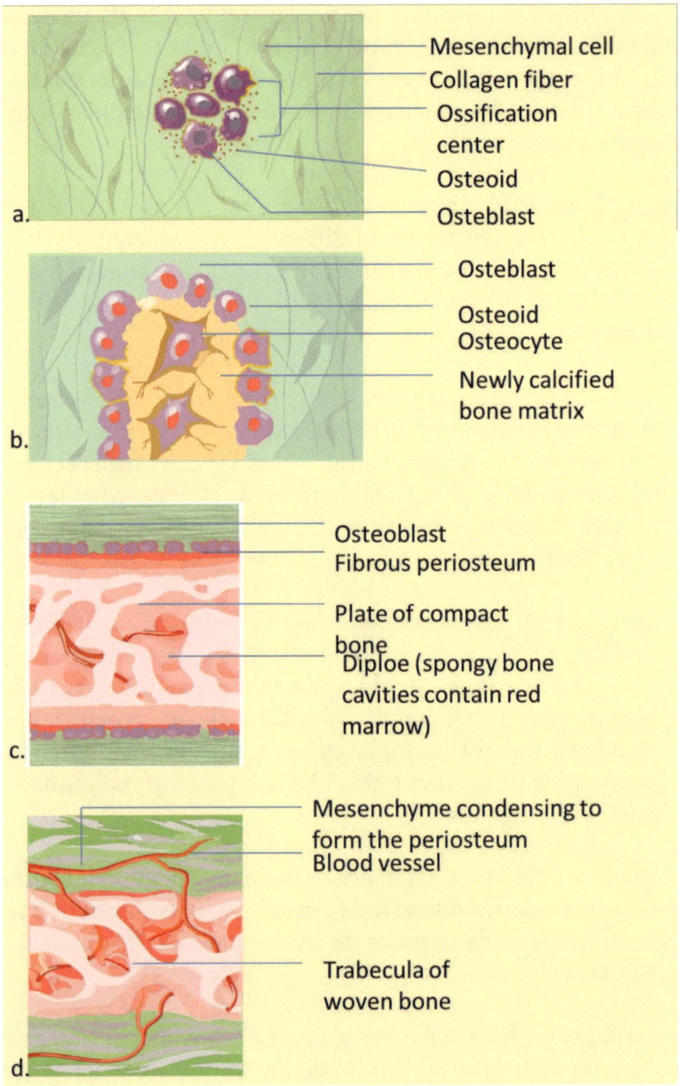

Figure 5.
The stage of intramembranous ossification. The following stages are (a) Mesenchymal cells group into clusters, and ossification centers form. (b) Secreted osteoid traps osteoblasts, which then become osteocytes. (c) Trabecular matrix and periosteum form. (d) Compact bone develops superficial to the trabecular bone, and crowded blood vessels condense into red marrow.

Bone tissue is divided into two, called the outer cortical and medullary regions, these two areas are destroyed by the resorption process; which goes along with further bone formation. The surrounding connective tissue will differentiate into the periosteum. The lining in the periosteum is rich in cells, has osteogenic function and contributes to the formation of thick bones as in the endosteum.

In adults, the bundle bone is usually only formed during rapid bone remodeling. This is reinforced by the presence of lamellar bone. Unlike bundle bone formation, lamellar bone development occurs only in mineralized matrix (e.g., cartilage that has calcified or bundle bone spicules). The nets in the bone bundle are filled to strengthen the lamellar bone, until compact bone is formed. Osteoblasts appear in the mineralized matrix, which then form a circle with intercellular matter surrounding the central vessels in several layers (Haversian system). Lamella bone is formed from 0.7 to 1.5 microns per day. The network is formed from complex fiber arrangements, responsible for its mechanical properties. The arrangement of apatites in the concentric layer of fibrils finally meets functional requirements. Lamellar bone depends on ongoing deposition and resorption which can be influenced by environmental factors, one of this which is orthodontic treatment.

4.1.2 Factors that influence intramembranous bone formation

Intramembranous bone formation from desmocranium (suture and periosteum) is mediated by mesenchymal skeletogenetic structures and is achieved through bone deposition and resorption [8]. This development is almost entirely controlled through local epigenetic factors and local environmental factors (i.e. by muscle strength, external local pressure, brain, eyes, tongue, nerves, and indirectly by endochondral ossification). Genetic factors only have a nonspecific morphogenetic effect on intramembranous bone formation and only determine external limits and increase the number of growth periods. Anomaly disorder (especially genetically produced) can affect endochondral bone formation, so local epigenetic factors and local environmental factors, including steps of orthodontic therapy, can directly affect intramembranous bone formation [3, 11].

4.2 Endochondral bone formation

During endochondral ossification, the tissue that will become bone is firstly formed from cartilage, separated from the joint and epiphysis, surrounded by perichondrium which then forms the periosteum [11]. Based on the location of mineralization, it can be divided into: Perichondral Ossification and Endochondral Ossification. Both types of ossification play an essential role in the formation of long bones where only endochondral ossification takes place in short bones. Perichondral ossification begins in the perichondrium. Mesenchymal cells from the tissue differentiate into osteoblasts, which surround bony diaphyseal before endochondral ossification, indirectly affect its direction [3, 8, 12]. Cartilage is transformed into bone is craniofacial bone that forms at the eigth prenatal week. Only bone on the cranial base and part of the skull bone derived from endochondral bone formation. Regarding to differentiate endochondral bone formation from chondrogenesis and intramembranous bone formation, five sequences of bone formation steps were determined [3].

4.2.1 The stages of endochondral bone formation

The statements below are the stages of endochondral bone formation (**Figure 6**) [4, 12]:

1. Mesenchymal cells group to form a shape template of the future bone.

2. Mesenchymal cells differentiate into chondrocytes (cartilage cells).

3. Hypertrophy of chondrocytes and calcified matrix with calcified central cartilage primordium matrix formed. Chondrocytes show hypertrophic changes and calcification from the cartilage matrix continues.

4. Entry of blood vessels and connective tissue cells. The nutrient artery supplies the perichondrium, breaks through the nutrient foramen at the mid-region and stimulates the osteoprogenitor cells in the perichondrium to produce

osteoblasts, which changes the perichondrium to the periosteum and starts the formation of ossification centers.

5. The periosteum continues its development and the division of cells (chondrocytes) continues as well, thereby increasing matrix production (this helps produce more length of bone).

6. The perichondrial membrane surrounds the surface and develops new chondroblasts.

7. Chondroblasts produce growth in width (appositional growth).

8. Cells at the center of the cartilage lyse (break apart) triggers calcification.

During endochondral bone formation, mesenchymal tissue firstly differentiates into cartilage tissue. Endochondral bone formation is morphogenetic adaptation (normal organ development) which produces continuous bone in certain areas that are prominently stressed. Therefore, this endochondral bone formation can be found in the bones associated with joint movements and some parts of the skull base. In hypertrophic cartilage cells, the matrix calcifies and the cells undergo degeneration. In cranial synchondrosis, there is proliferation in the formation of bones on both sides of the bone plate, this is distinguished by the formation of long bone epiphyses which only occurs on one side only [2, 14].

As the cartilage grows, capillaries penetrate it. This penetration initiates the transformation of the perichondrium into the bone-producing periosteum. Here, the osteoblasts form a periosteal collar of compact bone around the cartilage of the diaphysis. By the second or third month of fetal life, bone cell development and ossification ramps up and creates the **primary ossification center**, a region deep in the periosteal collar where ossification begins [4, 10].

While these deep changes occur, chondrocytes and cartilage continue to grow at the ends of the bone (the future epiphyses), which increase the bone length and at the same time bone also replaces cartilage in the diaphysis. By the time the fetal skeleton is fully formed, cartilage only remains at the joint surface as articular cartilage and between the diaphysis and epiphysis as the epiphyseal plate, the latter of which is responsible for the longitudinal growth of bones. After birth, this same sequence of events (matrix mineralization, death of chondrocytes, invasion of blood vessels from the periosteum, and seeding with osteogenic cells that become osteoblasts) occur in the epiphyseal regions, and each of these centers of activity is referred to as a **secondary ossification center** [4, 8, 10].

There are four important things about cartilage in endochondral bone formation:

1. Cartilage has a rigid and firm structure, but not usually calcified nature, giving three basic functions of growth (a) its flexibility can support an appropriate network structure (nose), (b) pressure tolerance in a particular place where compression occurs, (c) the location of growth in conjunction with enlarging bone (synchondrosis of the skull base and condyle cartilage).

2. Cartilage grows in two adjacent places (by the activity of the chondrogenic membrane) and grows in the tissues (chondrocyte cell division and the addition of its intercellular matrix).

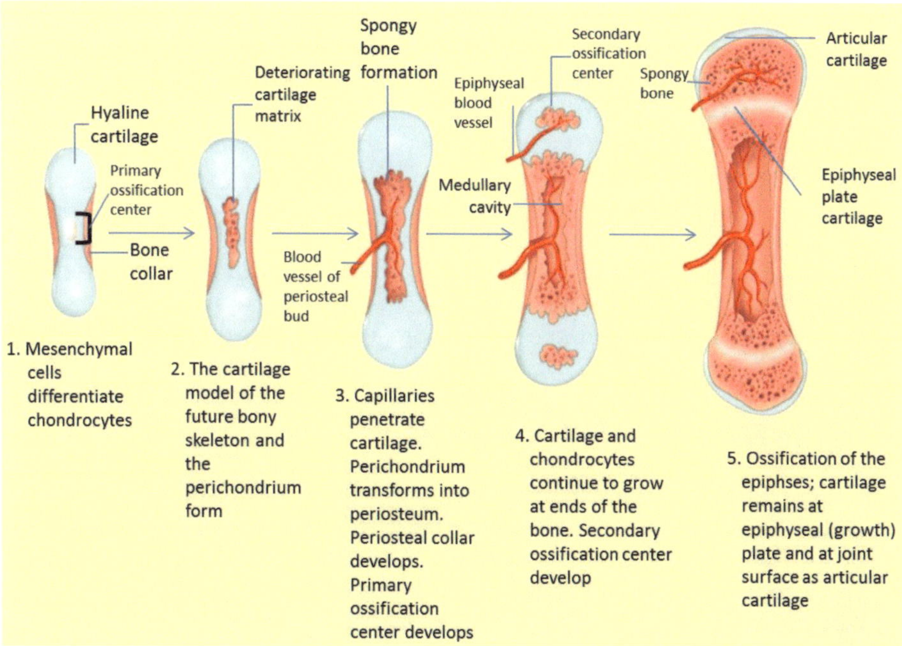

Figure 6.
The stage of endochondral ossification. The following stages are: (a) Mesenchymal cells differentiate into chondrocytes. (b) The cartilage model of the future bony skeleton and the perichondrium form. (c) Capillaries penetrate cartilage. Perichondrium transforms into periosteum. Periosteal collar develops. Primary ossification center develops. (d) Cartilage and chondrocytes continue to grow at ends of the bone. (e) Secondary ossification centers develop. (f) Cartilage remains at epiphyseal (growth) plate and at joint surface as articular cartilage.

3. Bone tissue is not the same as cartilage in terms of its tension adaptation and cannot grow directly in areas of high compression because its growth depends on the vascularization of bone formation covering the membrane.

4. Cartilage growth arises where linear growth is required toward the pressure direction, which allows the bone to lengthen to the area of strength and has not yet grown elsewhere by membrane ossification in conjunction with all periosteal and endosteal surfaces.

4.2.2 Factors that influence endochondral ossification

Membrane disorders or vascular supply problem of these essential membranes can directly result in bone cell death and ultimately bone damage. Calcified bones are generally hard and relatively inflexible and sensitive to pressure [12].

Cranial synchondrosis (e.g., spheno ethmoidal and spheno occipital growth) and endochondral ossification are further determined by chondrogenesis. Chondrogenesis is mainly influenced by genetic factors, similar to facial mesenchymal growth during initial embryogenesis to the differentiation phase of cartilage and cranial bone tissue.

This process is only slightly affected by local epigenetic and environmental factors. This can explain the fact that the cranial base is more resistant to deformation than desmocranium. Local epigenetic and environmental factors cannot trigger or inhibit the amount of cartilage formation. Both of these have little effect on the shape and direction of endochondral ossification. This has been analyzed especially during mandibular condyle growth.

Local epigenetics and environmental factors only affect the shape and direction of cartilage formation during endochondral ossification Considering the fact that condyle cartilage is a secondary cartilage, it is assumed that local factors provide a greater influence on the growth of mandibular condyle.

4.2.3 Chondrogenesis

Chondrogenesis is the process by which cartilage is formed from condensed mesenchyme tissue, which differentiates into chondrocytes and begins secreting the molecules that form the extracellular matrix [5, 14].

The statement below is five steps of chondrogenesis [8, 14]:

1. Chondroblasts produce a matrix: the extracellular matrix produced by cartilage cells, which is firm but flexible and capable of providing a rigid support.

2. Cells become embed in a matrix: when the chondroblast changes to be completely embed in its own matrix material, cartilage cells turn into chondrocytes. The new chondroblasts are distinguished from the membrane surface (perichondrium), this will result in the addition of cartilage size (cartilage can increase in size through apposition growth).

3. Chondrocytes enlarge, divide and produce a matrix. Cell growth continues and produces a matrix, which causes an increase in the size of cartilage mass from within. Growth that causes size increase from the inside is called interstitial growth.

4. The matrix remains uncalcified: cartilage matrix is rich of chondroitin sulfate which is associated with non-collagen proteins. Nutrition and metabolic waste are discharged directly through the soft matrix to and from the cell. Therefore, blood vessels aren't needed in cartilage.

5. The membrane covers the surface but is not essential: cartilage has a closed membrane vascularization called perichondrium, but cartilage can exist without any of these. This property makes cartilage able to grow and adapt where it needs pressure (in the joints), so that cartilage can receive pressure.

Endochondral ossification begins with characteristic changes in cartilage bone cells (hypertrophic cartilage) and the environment of the intercellular matrix (calcium laying), the formation which is called as primary spongiosa. Blood vessels and mesenchymal tissues then penetrate into this area from the perichondrium. The binding tissue cells then differentiate into osteoblasts and cells. Chondroblasts erode cartilage in a cave-like pattern (cavity). The remnants of mineralized cartilage the central part of laying the lamellar bone layer.

The osteoid layer is deposited on the calcified spicules remaining from the cartilage and then mineralized to form spongiosa bone, with fine reticular structures that resemble nets that possess cartilage fragments between the spicular bones. Spongy bones can turn into compact bones by filling empty cavities. Both endochondral and perichondral bone growth both take place toward epiphyses and joints. In the bone lengthening process during endochondral ossification depends on the growth of epiphyseal cartilage. When the epiphyseal line has been closed, the bone will not increase in length. Unlike bone, cartilage bone growth is based on apposition and interstitial growth. In areas where cartilage bone is covered by bone, various variations of zone characteristics, based on the developmental stages of each individual, can differentiate which then continuously merge with each other during the conversion process. Environmental influences (co: mechanism of orthopedic functional tools) have a strong effect on condylar cartilage because the bone is located more superficially [5].

5. Bone growth

Cartilage bone height development occurs during the third month of intra uterine life. Cartilage plate extends from the nasal bone capsule posteriorly to the foramen magnum at the base of the skull. It should be noted that cartilages which close to avascular tissue have internal cells obtained from the diffusion process from the outermost layer. This means that the cartilage must be flatter. In the early stages of development, the size of a very small embryo can form a chondroskeleton easily in which the further growth preparation occurs without internal blood supply [1].

During the fourth month in the uterus, the development of vascular elements to various points of the chondrocranium (and other parts of the early cartilage skeleton) becomes an ossification center, where the cartilage changes into an ossification center, and bone forms around the cartilage. Cartilage continues to grow rapidly but it is replaced by bone, resulting in the rapid increase of bone amount. Finally, the old chondrocranium amount will decrease in the area of cartilage and large portions of bone, assumed to be typical in ethmoid, sphenoid, and basioccipital bones. The cartilage growth in relation to skeletal bone is similar as the growth of the limbs [1, 3].

Longitudinal bone growth is accompanied by remodeling which includes appositional growth to thicken the bone. This process consists of bone formation and reabsorption. Bone growth stops around the age of 21 for males and the age of 18 for females when the epiphyses and diaphysis have fused (epiphyseal plate closure).

Normal bone growth is dependent on proper dietary intake of protein, minerals and vitamins. A deficiency of vitamin D prevents calcium absorption from the GI tract resulting in rickets (children) or osteomalacia (adults). Osteoid is produced but calcium salts are not deposited, so bones soften and weaken.

5.1 Oppositional bone growth

At the length of the long bones, the reinforcement plane appears in the middle and at the end of the bone, finally produces the central axis that is called the diaphysis and the bony cap at the end of the bone is called the epiphysis. Between epiphyses and diaphysis is a calcified area that is not calcified called the epiphyseal plate. Epiphyseal plate of the long bone cartilage is a major center for growth, and in fact, this cartilage is responsible for almost all the long growths of the bones. This is a layer of hyaline cartilage where ossification occurs in immature bones. On the epiphyseal side of the epiphyseal plate, the cartilage is formed. On the diaphyseal side, cartilage is ossified, and the diaphysis then grows in length. The epiphyseal plate is composed of five zones of cells and activity [3, 4].

Near the outer end of each epiphyseal plate is the active zone dividing the cartilage cells. Some of them, pushed toward diaphysis with proliferative activity, develop hypertrophy, secrete an extracellular matrix, and finally the matrix begins to fill with minerals and then is quickly replaced by bone. As long as cartilage cells multiply growth will continue. Finally, toward the end of the normal growth period, the rate of maturation exceeds the proliferation level, the latter of the cartilage is replaced by bone, and the epiphyseal plate disappears. At that time, bone growth is complete, except for surface changes in thickness, which can be produced by the periosteum [4]. Bones continue to grow in length until early adulthood. The lengthening is stopped in the end of adolescence which chondrocytes stop mitosis and plate thins out and replaced by bone, then diaphysis and epiphyses fuse to be one bone (**Figure 7**). The rate of growth is controlled by hormones. When the chondrocytes in the epiphyseal plate cease their proliferation and bone replaces the cartilage, longitudinal growth stops. All that remains of the epiphyseal plate is the epiphyseal line. Epiphyseal plate closure will occur in 18-year old females or 21-year old males.

5.1.1 Epiphyseal plate growth

The cartilage found in the epiphyseal gap has a defined hierarchical structure, directly beneath the secondary ossification center of the epiphysis. By close examination of the epiphyseal plate, it appears to be divided into five zones (starting from the epiphysis side) (**Figure 8**) [4]:

1. The resting zone: it contains hyaline cartilage with few chondrocytes, which means no morphological changes in the cells.

2. The proliferative zone: chondrocytes with a higher number of cells divide rapidly and form columns of stacked cells parallel to the long axis of the bone.

3. The hypertrophic cartilage zone: it contains large chondrocytes with cells increasing in volume and modifying the matrix, effectively elongating bone

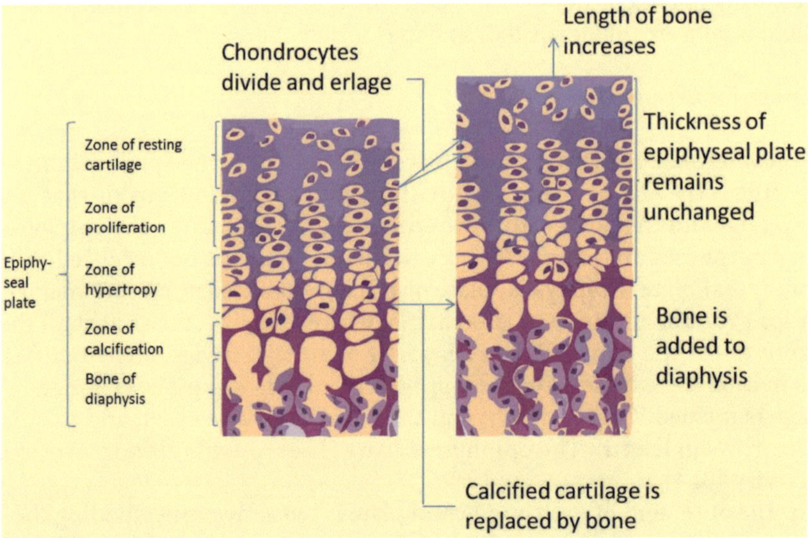

Figure 7.
Oppositional bone growth and remodeling. The epiphyseal plate is responsible for longitudinal bone growth.

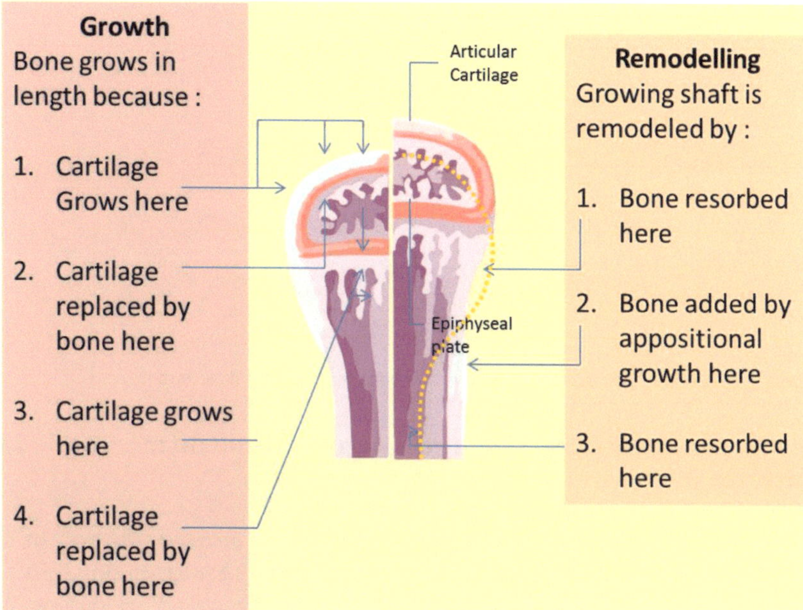

Figure 8.
Epiphyseal plate growth. Five zones of epiphyseal growth plate includes: 1. resting zone, 2. proliferation zone, 3. hypertrophic cartilage zone, 4. calcified cartilage zone, and 5. ossification zone.

whose cytoplasm has accumulated glycogen. The resorbed matrix is reduced to thin septa between the chondrocytes.

4. The calcified cartilage zone: chondrocytes undergo apoptosis, the thin septa of cartilage matrix become calcified.

5. The ossification zone: endochondral bone tissue appears. Blood capillaries and osteoprogenitor cells (from the periosteum) invade the cavities left by the chondrocytes. The osteoprogenitor cells form osteoblasts, which deposit bone matrix over the three-dimensional calcified cartilage matrix.

5.2 Appositional bone growth

When bones are increasing in length, they are also increasing in diameter; diameter growth can continue even after longitudinal growth stops. This is called appositional growth. The bone is absorbed on the endosteal surface and added to the periosteal surface. Osteoblasts and osteoclasts play an essential role in appositional bone growth where osteoblasts secrete a bone matrix to the external bone surface from diaphysis, while osteoclasts on the diaphysis endosteal surface remove bone from the internal surface of diaphysis. The more bone around the medullary cavity is destroyed, the more yellow marrow moves into empty space and fills space. Osteoclasts resorb the old bone lining the medullary cavity, while osteoblasts through intramembrane ossification produce new bone tissue beneath the periosteum. Periosteum on the bone surface also plays an important role in increasing thickness and in reshaping the external contour. The erosion of old bone along the medullary cavity and new bone deposition under the periosteum not only increases the diameter of the diaphysis but also increases the diameter of the medullary cavity. This process is called modeling (**Figure 9**) [3, 4, 15].

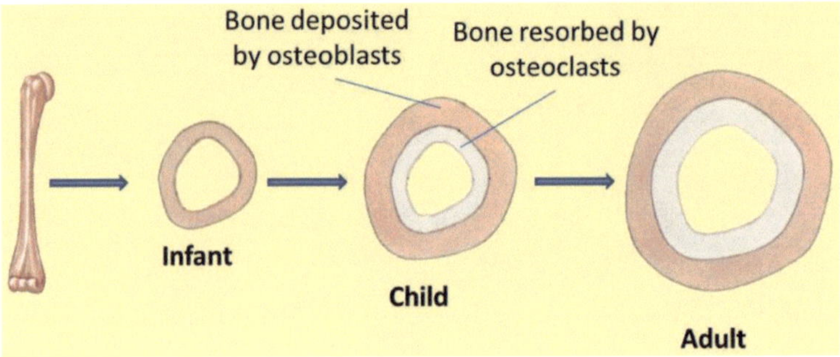

Figure 9.
Appositional bone growth. Bone deposit by osteoblast as bone resorption by osteoclast.

6. The role of mesenchymal stem cell migration and differentiation in bone formation

Recent research reported that bone microstructure is also the principle of bone function, which regulates its mechanical function. Bone tissue function influenced by many factors, such as hormones, growth factors, and mechanical loading. The microstructure of bone tissue is distribution and alignment of biological apatite (BAp) crystallites. This is determined by the direction of bone cell behavior, for example cell migration and cell regulation. Ozasa et al. found that artificial control the direction of mesenchymal stem cell (MSCs) migration and osteoblast alignment can reconstruct bone microstructure, which guide an appropriate bone formation during bone remodeling and regeneration [16].

Bone development begins with the replacement of collagenous mesenchymal tissue by bone. Generally, bone is formed by endochondral or intramembranous ossification. Intramembranous ossification is essential in the bone such as skull, facial bones, and pelvis which MSCs directly differentiate to osteoblasts. While, endochondral ossification plays an important role in most bones in the human skeleton, including long, short, and irregular bones, which MSCs firstly experience to condensate and then differentiate into chondrocytes to form the cartilage growth plate and the growth plate is then gradually replaced by new bone tissue [3, 8, 12].

MSC migration and differentiation are two important physiological processes in bone formation. MSCs migration raise as an essential step of bone formation because MSCs initially need to migrate to the bone surface and then contribute in bone formation process, although MSCs differentiation into osteogenic cells is also crucial. MSC migration during bone formation has attracted more attention. Some studies show that MSC migration to the bone surface is crucial for bone formation [17]. Bone marrow and periosteum are the main sources of MSCs that participate in bone formation [18].

In the intramembranous ossification, MSCs undergo proliferation and differentiation along the osteoblastic lineage to form bone directly without first forming cartilage. MSC and preosteoblast migration is involved in this process and are mediated by plentiful factors in vivo and in vitro. MSCs initially differentiate into preosteoblasts which proliferate near the bone surface and secrete ALP. Then they become mature osteoblasts and then form osteocytes which embedded in an extracellular matrix (ECM). Other factors also regulate the intramembranous ossification of MSCs such as Runx2, special AT-rich sequence binding protein 2 (SATB 2), and Osterix as well as pathways, like the wnt/β-catenin pathway and bone morphogenetic protein (BMP) pathway [17, 19].

In the endochondral ossification, MSCs are first condensed to initiate cartilage model formation. The process is mediated by BMPs through phosphorylating and activating receptor SMADs to transduce signals. During condensation, the central part of MSCs differentiates into chondrocytes and secretes cartilage matrix. While, other cells in the periphery, form the perichondrium that continues expressing type I collagen and other important factors, such as proteoglycans and ALP. Chondrocytes undergo rapid proliferation. Chondrocytes in the center become maturation, accompanied with an invasion of hypertrophic cartilage by the vasculature, followed by differentiation of osteoblasts within the perichondrium and marrow cavity. The inner perichondrium cells differentiate into osteoblasts, which secrete bone matrix to form the bone collar after vascularization in the hypertrophic cartilage. Many factors that regulate endochondral ossification are growth factors (GFs), transforming growth factor-β (TGF-β), Sry-related high-mobility group box 9 (Sox9) and Cell-to-cell interaction [17, 19].

7. Conclusions

- Osteogenesis/ossification is the process in which new layers of bone tissue are placed by osteoblasts.

- During bone formation, woven bone (haphazard arrangement of collagen fibers) is remodeled into lamellar bones (parallel bundles of collagen in a layer known as lamellae)

- Periosteum is a connective tissue layer on the outer surface of the bone; the endosteum is a thin layer (generally only one layer of cell) that coats all the internal surfaces of the bone

- Major cell of bone include: osteoblasts (from osteoprogenitor cells, forming osteoid that allow matrix mineralization to occur), osteocytes (from osteoblasts; closed to lacunae and retaining the matrix) and osteoclasts (from hemopoietic lineages; locally erodes matrix during bone formation and remodeling.

- The process of bone formation occurs through two basic mechanisms:
    - Intramembranous bone formation occurs when bone forms inside the mesenchymal membrane. Bone tissue is directly laid on primitive connective tissue referred to mesenchyma without intermediate cartilage involvement. It forms bone of the skull and jaw; especially only occurs during development as well as the fracture repair.
    - Endochondral bone formation occurs when hyaline cartilage is used as a precursor to bone formation, then bone replaces hyaline cartilage, forms and grows all other bones, occurs during development and throughout life.

- During interstitial epiphyseal growth (elongation of the bone), the growth plate with zonal organization of endochondral ossification, allows bone to lengthen without epiphyseal growth plates enlarging zones include:
    - Zone of resting.
    - Zone of proliferation.
    - Zone of hypertrophy.

    - Zone of calcification.
    - Zone of ossification and resorption.

- During appositional growth, osteoclasts resorb old bone that lines the medullary cavity, while osteoblasts, via intramembranous ossification, produce new bone tissue beneath the periosteum.
- Mesenchymal stem cell migration and differentiation are two important physiological processes in bone formation.

Acknowledgements

The author is grateful to Zahrona Kusuma Dewi for assistance with preparation of the manuscript.

Conflict of interest

The authors declare that there is no conflict of interests regarding the publication of this paper.

Acronyms and abbreviations

ALP	alkaline phosphatase
Bap	biological apatite
BMP	bone morphogenetic protein
ECM	extracellular matrix
GFs	growth factors
MSCs	mesenchymal stem cells
Runx2	runt-related transcription factor 2
SATB 2	special AT-rich sequence binding protein 2
Sox9	sry-related high-mobility group box 9
TGF-β	transforming growth factor-β

Author details

Rosy Setiawati* and Paulus Rahardjo
Department of Radiology, Faculty of Medicine Airlangga University, Dr. Soetomo General Hospital, Surabaya, East Java, Indonesia

*Address all correspondence to: dr_setia76@yahoo.co.id

References

[1] Vanputte CL, Regan JL, Russo AF. Skeletal system: Bones and joints. In: Seeley's Essentials of Anatomy & Physiology. 8th ed. USA: Mc Graw Hill; 2013. pp. 110-149

[2] Muscolino JE. Kinesiology the Skelatal System and Muscle Function. 2nd ed. New York: Elsevier Inc.; 2011

[3] Cashman KD, Ginty F. Bone. New York: Elsevier; 2003. pp. 1106-1112

[4] OpenStax College. Anatomy & Physiology. Texas: Rice University; 2013. pp. 203-231

[5] Florencia-Silva R, Rodrigues G, Sasso-Cerri E, Simoes MJ, Cerri PS. Biology of bone tissue: Structure, function, and factors that influence bone cells. Biolmed Research International. 2015:1-17

[6] Tim A. Bone Structure and Bone Remodelling. London: University College London; 2014

[7] Mohamed AM. Review article an overview of bone cells and their regulating. Malaysian Journal of Medical Sciences. 2008;**15**(1):4-12

[8] Akter F, Ibanez J. Bone and cartilage tissue engineering. In: Akter F, editor. Tissue Engineering Made Easy [Internet]. 1st ed. New York: Elsevier Inc.; 2016. pp. 77-98. DOI: 10.1016/B978-0-12-805361-4.00008-4

[9] Guus van der Bie MD, editor. Morphological Anatomy from a Phenomenological Point of View. Rome: Louis Bolk Institute; 2012

[10] Wojnar R. Bone and Cartilage–Its Structure and Physical Properties. Weinheim: Wiley-VCH Verlag GmbH & Co.; 2010

[11] Karaplis AC. Embryonic development of bone and regulation of intramembranous and endochondral bone formation. In: Bilezikian J, Raisz L, Martin TJ, editors. Principles of Bone Biology. 3rd ed. New York: Academic Press; 2008. pp. 53-84

[12] Dennis SC, Berkland CJ, Bonewald LF, Determore MS. Endochondral ossification for enhancing bone regeneration: Converging native ECM biomaterials and developmental engineering in vivo. Tissue Engineering. Part B, Reviews. 2015;**21**(3):247-266

[13] Clarke B. Normal bone anatomy and physiology. Clinical Journal of the American Society of Nephrology. 2008;**3**:131-139

[14] Provot S, Schipani E, Wu JY, Kronenberg H. Development of the skeleton. In: Marcus R, Dempster D, Cauley J, Feldman D, editors. Osteoporosis [Internet]. 4th ed. New York: Elsevier; 2013. pp. 97-126. DOI: 10.1016/B978-0-12-415853-5.00006-6

[15] Schindeler A, Mcdonald MM, Bokko P, Little DG. Bone remodeling during fracture repair: The cellular picture. Seminars in Cell & Developmental Biology. 2008;**19**:459-466. DOI. 10.1016/j.semcdb.2008.07.004

[16] Ozasa R, Matsugaki A, Isobe Y, Saku T, Yun H-S, Nakano T. Construction of human induced pluripotent stem cell-derived oriented bone matrix microstructure by using in vitro engineered anisotropic culture model. Journal of Biomedial Materials Research Part A. 2018;**106**:360-369

[17] Su P, Tian Y, Yang C, Ma X, Wang X. Mesenchymal stem cell migration during bone formation and bone diseases therapy. International Journal of Molecular Sciences. 2018;**19**:2343

[18] Wang X, Wang Y, Gou W, Lu Q. Role of mesenchymal stem cells in bone regeneration and fracture repair: A review. International Orthopaedics. 2013;**37**:2491-2498

[19] Fakhry M, Hamade E, Badran B, Buchet R, Magne D. Molecular mechanisms of mesenchymal stem cell differentiation towards osteoblasts. World Journal of Stem Cells. 2013;**5**(4):136-148

Chapter 2

Wnt Signaling and Genetic Bone Diseases

Yanqin Lu and Jinxiang Han

Abstract

The Wnt signal transduction plays a vital role in regulating development throughout the animal kingdom. The Wnt signal transduction is complex, including Wnt ligands, receptors, coreceptors, transducers, transcription factors, antagonists, agonists and their modulators, and target genes. It is classified into β-catenin-dependent canonical and independent non-canonical Wnt (mainly planar cell polarity and Wnt/Ca^{2+}) signaling pathways. Wnt signaling pathway is causative to multiple human diseases. Gene mutations from the components of WNT signaling machinery have been identified to relate with low or high bone mass diseases, such as osteogenesis imperfecta, Robinow syndrome, osteoporosis-pseudoglioma syndrome, and sclerosteosis. In this review, we provide an update of the Wnt signaling pathway and the bone diseases caused by the aberrant components of the pathways.

Keywords: Wnt, Wnt signaling pathway, genetic bone diseases

1. Introduction

The Wnt1 gene (originally named Int1) was identified in 1982 as a gene activated by integration of mouse mammary tumor virus (MMTV) proviral DNA in virally induced breast tumors [1]. The Int1 proto-oncogene is highly conserved in many species, the fly wingless (Wg) gene in Drosophila, functions in controlling segment polarity during larval development and also activated in cancer, was found to be a homolog of Wnt1 [2]. Later, McMahon and Moon found that ectopic expression of Int1 in Xenopus leads to dual axis formation, when mouse Int1 RNA was injected into Xenopus embryos. Duplication of axial structures was abolished by substitution of a single, conserved cysteine residue of Int1 [3]. Later, more and more Wnt family members were identified.

2. Wnt and its secretion

2.1 Wnt proteins and their structure

Till now, Wnt family currently includes 19 secreted lipid-modified glycoproteins in most mammalian genomes, including the human genome. They fall into 12 conserved Wnt subfamilies, of which at least 11 of these occur in the genome of a Cnidaria, highlighting the vital role of Wnt family members in the process of organismal patterning throughout the animal kingdom [4]. In humans, Wnt1 and Wnt10b are located adjacent to each other on chromosome 12, and they are

IntechOpen

transcribed in opposite directions. Wnt6 and Wnt10a are located adjacent to each other on chromosome 2 and transcribed from the same strand of DNA. Other Wnt genes are prone to be clustered within the human genome also, including Wnt2 and Wnt16, Wnt3a and Wnt14, and Wnt3 and Wnt15 [5]. Wnt1-Wnt6-Wnt10 is an ancient cluster of Wnt genes in a common ancestor of vertebrates and arthropods and this cluster was duplicated leading to Wnt1-Wnt6-Wnt10a and Wnt1-Wnt6-Wnt10b cluster in vertebrates [5]. Based on their ability to induce transformation of the epithelial cell line C57MG, Wnt family are classified into highly transformation members, which includes Wnt1, Wnt2, Wnt3, and Wnt3a, and nontransformation members including Wnt4, Wnt5a, Wnt5b, and Wnt7b. High transformation members are related to Wnt/β-catenin canonical pathway and nontransformation members are related to noncanonical Wnt pathways. Wnt6 and Wnt7a are categorized as intermediate transformation members, leading to weak morphological changes [6].

Wnt genes encode proteins of ~350–400 residues in length, with molecular weight of about 40 kDa in size. Little is known about the structure of Wnts for their highly hydrophobic characteristics. In 2012, the 3D structure of Xenopus Wnt8 protein as bound to mouse Frizzled-8 cysteine-rich domain (CRD) was solved. XWnt8 is consist of an N-terminal α-helical domain (NTD) that includes the lipid-modified thumb and a C-terminal cysteine-rich region (CTD). They resemble the extended thumb and index fingers to project into a pocket in the opposite side of Fzd-CRD [7].

2.2 Posttranslational modifications of Wnts in the ER and Golgi apparatus

Wnt proteins share some features in common. They have an amino-terminal signal peptide that targets them to the ER and undergo a series of posttranslational modifications in the secretory pathway before transporting into the extracellular space. Wnts contain several charged residues and 23–25 cysteines on average, and some of them participate in inter- and intramolecular disulfide bonds, leading to Wnt folding and multimerization [7, 8]. All Wnt proteins (except Drosophila WntD) undergo posttranslational acylation and glycosylation [9]. There are two conserved residues of fatty acylation reported till now. The first acylation is palmitate attached to a conserved cysteine residue 77 in murine Wnt3a through a thioester linkage. The second lipid modification was identified at the position of serine 209 in murine Wnt3a protein. This conserved residue is modified by a monounsaturated fatty acid, palmitoleic acid [10–12]. This lipid posttranslational modification leads to extremely hydrophobicity of Wnts and restrict Wnt proteins to membranes by injecting into the lipid bilayer [9, 11]. Cys77 mutant leads to the loss of Wnt3a activity without affecting secretion, while Wnt3a Ser209Ala mutant is retained in the ER and secretion is blocked [10, 11]. Crystal structure of XWnt8 discovered that only conserved serine (corresponding to serine 209 in murine Wnt3a) is acylated. Cys77 is involved in the formation of disulfide bond with a second conserved cysteine [7]. Till now, *Drosophila* WntD is the only nonlipidated member of Wnt family [13]. Monoacylation is further corroborated by the lack of Cys77 palmitoylation study [14, 15]. This serine acylation is essential for Wnt binding to the coreceptor Frizzled, Wnt secretion and binding to the chaperone Wntless [7, 16, 17].

The attachment of palmitoleate to Wnt's conserved serine is mediated through substrate specificity by acyltransferase Porcupine, which is homologous to the superfamily of acyltransferase enzymes localized to the endoplasmic reticulum (ER). Mutation of Porcupine impeded Wnt acylation activity in vitro [18]. Wnt palmitoylation is reversible and it can be removed by Notum, the serine hydrolase, and this deacylase activity is specific for Wnt proteins [19, 20]. Hence, Notum's inhibitors have potential for treating degenerative diseases by targeting Wnt signaling [21].

N-Glycosylation is another common posttranslational modification of Wnt ligands, and nitrogen atom of multiple asparagine residues of Wnts is attached to oligosaccharide. This modification precedes palmitoylation and is independent of it [22, 23]. The number and position of N-glycosylation vary in different Wnt members [24]. The role of Wnt protein's N-glycosylation is unclear, but usually, it influences secretion, but not folding and structure [9]. For Wg protein, which has two known N-glycosylation, Asn103 and Asn414, Wg mutant can activate downstream signaling in both autocrine and paracrine signaling, despite reduced secretion ability. Loss of N-glycosylation of Wnt1 impairs paracrine signaling. For Wnt3a and Wnt5a, N-glycosylation is essential for secretion, but not for the activity of Wnt5a protein [23, 25]. Porcupine plays an important role in both lipid and glycosylated modifications of Wnts and its mutant displayed a decreased N-glycosylation activity [8–10, 26].

Besides acylation and N-glycosylation of Wnt proteins, several other modifications are included in the posttranslational modification. Posttranslational tyrosine sulfation of Wnt5a and Wnt11 is essential for the formation of Wnt5a/Wnt11 complexes, which induce the efficient signaling in the context of Xenopus axis formation [27]. Wnt1 is attached to glycosylphosphatidylinositol (GPI) anchor on the leaflet of the plasma membrane by the glycolipid tail. PGAP1 gene participates in this modification by creating a hydrophobic Wnt1 that is retained in the ER [28].

2.3 Secretion and release of Wnt proteins

After posttranslational palmitoylation and N-glycosylation, mature Wnt proteins are then transported from the Golgi to the plasma membrane for secretion by the conserved multipass transmembrane Wntless (Wls) receptor (known as GPR177 in mammals) [29]. Wnt secretion could not proceed with the absence of Wls, but other signaling proteins are not influenced by the removal of Wls [30–32]. Wls knockout mice exhibit impairment of body axis formation, and a phenotype mimics the deficiency of Wnt3. Wls is activated by β-catenin and LEF/TCF-dependent transcription and its mutants impede Wnt secretion and signaling [33]. Wls is essential for Wnt signaling, and tissue-specific knockouts of Wls impede varieties of processes including bone mass, skin homeostasis, peripheral lung differentiation, and pulmonary vascular development [34–36].

Endogenous Wls contains a carboxy-terminal ER-targeting signal, which directs Wls localizing predominantly in the ER, where it binds with acylated Wnt proteins [16, 37]. P24 protein family, which acts as cargo receptor for Wnt in the early secretory pathway, is essential for proper export of Wg from the ER [38–40]. Sec22 is packaged together with Wg and p24 during the early secretory phase of Wg and it functions as the vesicle SNARE (soluble NSF attachment protein receptor) [40].

The detailed mechanisms for Wnt secretion are not clear. Wnts-Wls complex transport from ER to plasma membrane is COPII vesicles dependent. Once arriving at the plasm membrane, Wnt is then released from plasm membrane and binds to lipoprotein particles or heparin sulfate proteoglycans (HSPGs) [41, 42]. The other theory supports that Wnt-Wls complex keeps together and internalizes at plasm membrane and dissociates from each other in endosomes. Then, Wnts is released through a recycling endosomal pathway and Wls is transported back to TGN through a retromer-dependent pathway [42–44]. Dpy23 and Vps35 are reported to regulate recycling of *C. elegans* Mig-14, which is the homolog of Wls. Wls is restricted to the plasma membrane with the Dyp23 mutant [45]. Retromer complex consists of Vps35, Vps29, Vps26, Vps10, Vps5, and Vps17 in yeast [46–48]. Vps35, Vps29, and Vps26 subcomplexes mediate cargo recognition and retrieve Vps10p from endosomes to the Golgi [47]. Vps35 mutant has no influence on the transportation of Wls to plasm membrane and endocytosis, but the retromer-dependent shuttle to the Golgi is inaccessible, and endocytosed Wls progresses to MVBs and lysosomes for degradation [43, 44, 49]. Vps5 and Vps17 are membrane-bound subcomplexes of retromer, and they are sorting nexins (SNX) with a phosphoinositide-binding SNX-phox homology (SNX-PX) domain [50]. Nexins SNX1, SNX2, SNX5, and SNX6 are SNX-BAR coat complex that interact with cargo-selective Vps35-Vps29-Vps26 complex. They are needed for most of the retromer cargo proteins, but not for the process of Wls recycling [50, 51]. Wls recycling specifically relies on SNX3, the retromer without BAR domain [51, 52]. SNX3 cointeracts with Wls and Vps26 on early endosomes and helps the association of the cargo-selective complex to Wls [51]. Wls recycled in Golgi further retrogrades transport to ER, which is mediated by the conserved C terminal sequence of Wls targeting ER. This process is currently COPI dependent and requires ER-Golgi intermediate compartment ERGIC2, though retrieval mechanisms need further investigation [37, 53]. Recently, miR-307a is found to inhibit Wg secretion by targeting Wls, and its overexpression induces ER stress specifically in the Wg-expressing cells. KKVY motif of Wg is responsible for its retrieval and ER stress [53].

Wnts are classic morphogens, which play an important role in tissue patterning by activating their target genes in a concentration-dependent manner and act in short and long range way [14, 54]. Various carriers have been identified that associate with extracellular Wnts, which include exovesicles [55], exosomes [56, 57], lipoprotein [41, 58], cytonemes (filopodia-like protrusions) [59–61], and Swim (secreted Wnt-interacting molecule) belonging to lipocalin family of protein [62]. These secreted Wnts associate to specific receptors on target cells to activate either canonical Wnt/β-catenin pathway or noncanonical Wnt/Ca^{2+} pathway.

3. Wnt signaling pathway

3.1 The canonical Wnt signaling pathway

The Wnt signaling pathway serves many important functions in body axis patterning, embryonic development, cell proliferation, and differentiation. In the absence of Wnt signaling, β-catenin is phosphorylated and ubiquitinated to keep low level by forming β-catenin destruction complex. The complex includes β-catenin, axin, casein kinase-1 (CK1), glycogen synthase kinase-3β (GSK-3β), and the adenomatous polyposis coli (APC) [63, 64]. PP2A and HSP105 are also involved in this complex. HSP105 recruits the phosphatase PP2A to the degradation complex to antagonize the phosphorylation of β-catenin, thus keeping the balance of phosphorylation-dephosphorylation [65]. Maintaining a phosphostatus balance of the β-catenin protein leads to its accumulation or degradation based on the signaling cues. The complex binds and phosphorylates β-catenin, leading to the ubiquitination by β-transducin repeat-containing protein (β-TrCP) ubiquitin ligase and subsequent proteasomal degradation [66].

In the presence of Wnt ligands, Wnt ligands bind to the specific receptor including Frizzled (Fzd) family member and subsequent LRP5/6 coreceptor. Axin is dephosphorylated and sequestered at the membrane. The binding triggers the recruitment of phosphoprotein disheveled (Dsh/Dvl) to form the LRP/Fzd/Dsh complexes, inducing the phosphorylation of LRP by CK1ϒ and GSK3; as a consequence, axin is then dephosphorylated and sequestered at the membrane and destruction complex is inactivated. The signalosome composed of Fzd, LRP5/6, Dvl, axin, GSK3, and CK1 destroys the β-catenin destruction complex [67, 68].

Hence, cytosolic β-catenin accumulates and localizes to the nucleus, where it interacts with TCF/LEF family members and recruits other transcriptional coactivators, such as CBP, TBP, and BRG-1, to induce target gene expression [69, 70].

Axin is a scaffold protein and acts as an anchor for other four proteins in the complex. In addition, axin participates in the LRP6 phosphorylation on the PPPSPxS motifs, which in turn cause the accumulation of axin in the destruction complex and then lead to the initiation of β-catenin signaling [71]. Recently, axin was found to be fully phosphorylated in the state of Wnt-off and partly phosphorylated in the state of Wnt-on mediated by GSK-3β [72].

The role of APC in Wnt signaling is complex and multiple. APC acts as a carrier for GSK-3β and axin that promotes phosphorylation and consequent ubiquitin-dependent degradation of β-catenin [73]. It binds to β-catenin by 15 or 20-mer amino acid repeats. APC promotes export of β-catenin from nucleus, and hence the expression and transcriptional activity of nuclear β-catenin are reduced indirectly [74]. Meanwhile, APC downregulates the β-catenin/TCF transcription by directly interacting with transcriptional repressor C-terminal binding protein (CtBP) [75, 76]. APC may also serve as a positive regulator for Wnt signaling through downregulation of axin [77]. APC is vital for the phosphorylation of axin in both Wnt-off and Wnt-on states, the association with activated phospho-LRP6 and the rapid transition in axin activity [72]. Phosphorylated β-catenin requires APC for its targeting to ubiquitin ligase and protection from dephosphorylation mediated by protein phosphatase 2A (PP2A) [78]. Recently, APC was found to impede clathrin-dependent signalosome formation in the absence of ligand [79].

GSK3-β and CK1 are both serine/threonine kinases that phosphorylate the N-terminal portion of cytosolic β-catenin, and phosphorylation of β-catenin begins at Ser45 by CK1α and then phosphorylation of residues Thr41, Ser37, and Ser33 [80, 81]. Meanwhile, CK1, perhaps also GSK3β, phosphorylates APC on the 20-mer repeats. Phosphorylation of APC increases the binding affinity to β-catenin, and β-catenin disassociates from axin [63]. Phosphorylated β-catenin is then recognized by β-TrCP1, an F-box protein component of an Skp1/Cul1/F-box (SCF)-type ubiquitin ligase complex [82], followed by recruitment of E3 ubiquitin ligase and degraded by the 26S proteasome [83].

PP2A is a cellular heterotrimeric serine-threonine protein phosphatase consisting of a structural (A), a regulatory (B), and a catalytic subunit (C) [84]. PP2A has a dual opposite regulation role for Wnt signaling. PP2A is regarded as one of the members of β-catenin degradation complex [85]. PP2A dephosphorylates GSK3β through recruitment of DNAJB6 (DnaJ homolog subfamily B member 6) and HSPA8 (heat-shock cognate protein, HSC70) [86]. The B56 subunit of PP2A interacts with N-terminal of APC and decreases the amount of β-catenin and inhibits transcription of its target genes [87, 88]. Also, B56ε is required for Wnt/β-catenin signaling downstream of the Wnt ligand and upstream of Dsh [89]. PR61 β regulates Wnt signaling by inhibiting Dvl- and β-catenin–dependent T-cell factor activation, or suppressing the downstream target genes [90]. PR55α subunit of PP2A acts as the positive regulator for Wnt signaling. It interacts with β-catenin directly and controls dephosphorylation and degradation of β-catenin. Knockdown of PR55α increases β-catenin phosphorylation and decreases Wnt signaling, whereas is the same as PR55α overexpression [91, 92]. PP2C also upregulates Wnt signaling through the dephosphorylation of axin [93]. Meanwhile, many subunits of PP2A, such as PR55α, A, C, B56α, and PR61β and ϒ, are reported to interact with axin [87, 90, 91]. PR61ε subunit of PP2A is involved in the initiation of the Wnt pathway. PR61ε binds to Fzd receptor, and binding of Wnt ligands promote the interaction of LRP5/6-associated CK1ε and PR61ε. The latter dephosphatases CK1ε, leading to recruitment of Dvl-2 to the receptor complex and the initiation of the Wnt signaling [94].

3.2 The noncanonical Wnt pathway

Due to varieties of both Wnts and their receptors and coreceptors, Wnt pathways are multiple and complex. There are multiple branches of β-catenin–independent Wnt signaling pathways. One is the Wnt/Ca^{2+} pathway, modulating intracellular Ca^{2+} level. The second is the Wnt/planar cell polarity (PCP) pathway, utilizing small Rho-like GTPases [95].

3.2.1 Wnt/PCP pathway

Polarization is a global property of cells and tissues. In addition to the ubiquitous epithelial apical-basal axis, many multicellular tissues also have planar cell polarity, orthology to apico-basal polarity [96, 97]. Compared with canonical Wnt signaling, various cell surface receptors have been involved in PCP signaling. PCP is composed of core protein complexes and Fat/Dachsous (Ds)/Fj (four-jointed) group. The latter is reported to act upstream of PCP to provide a directional information [98, 99]. Core protein complexes are composed of Frizzled, Flamingo (Fmi/Celsr), Van Gogh (*Drosophila* Vang or Stb/mammalian Vang), disheveled (Dsh/Dvl), Diego, and Prickle (Pk) [100]. The core complex within puncta is predominately stable than elsewhere in the junctions and highly asymmetrically organized, while core protein stoichiometry in both puncta and nonpuncta region is similar. The core protein is assembled around a stoichiometric Fz-Fmi nucleus. The amount of Fz and Stb is maintained relative to their binding partners for normal asymmetry [101]. In many cancers, Wnt/PCP signaling is upregulated and it contributes to cancer malignancy by enhancing the proliferation and migration, priming metastasis niches, and causing resistance to therapy [102, 103].

3.2.2 Wnt/Ca^{2+} signaling pathway

Wnt5a is the most common ligand for noncanonical Wnt signal transducer. It activates calcium signaling pathway by binding to receptor Fz2, 3, 4, 5, and Fz6, as well as coreceptor Ror1/2, which is the membrane-bound receptor tyrosine kinase [104-107]. Dvl, axin, and GSK organize the complex and GSK phosphorylates Ror coreceptor [108]. Wnt/Fz/Ror then activates phospholipase C (PLC), leading to the generation of diacylglycerol (DAG) and inositol 1,4,5-trisphosphate (IP3) from membrane-bound phospholipid phosphatidyl inositol 4,5-bisphosphate (PIP2). Recently, SEC1413/the Sec14-like protein acts as GTPase proteins to mediate specific Wnt-Fz-Dvl complex signals downstream to phospholipase C δ4a (PLCδ4a). The binding of SEC141 to Wnt-Fz-Dvl complexes induces its translocation of SEC1413 to the plasma membrane, and then further binds to and activates PLCδ4a. In turn, PLCδ4a acts as a GTPase-activating protein to promote the hydrolysis of Sec14l3-bound GTP to GDP [109]. IP3 promotes the concentration of intracellular Ca^{2+}, which activates calcineurin, phospho-serine/threonine specific protein phosphatase and calcium calmodulin-dependent protein kinase II (CaMKII). In turn, nuclear factor associated with T cells (NFAT) and regulatory proteins NFkB are activated. DAG activates protein kinase C (PKC), which further activates NFkB and CREB. Meanwhile, Wnt/Fz interaction may activate phosphodiesterase 6 (PDE6) in a calcium-dependent manner, leading to a decrease in cyclic guanosine monophosphate (cGMP) [110].

4. Wnt signaling in genetic bone diseases

Both bone modeling and remodeling are regulated by Wnt signaling, and mutation of Wnt signaling components is linked to various genetic bone diseases. **Table 1**

Phenotype	Phenotype MIM number	Inheritance	Gene	Gene MIM number	Reference
Wnt ligands					
Osteogenesis imperfecta, type XV	615220	AR	Wnt1	164820	Pyott et al. [125]
Osteoporosis, early-onset, susceptibility to, autosomal dominant	615221		Wnt1		Laine et al. [127]
Tetraamelia syndrome 1	273395	AR	Wnt3	165330	Niemann et al. [115]
Robinow syndrome, autosomal dominant 1	180700	AD	Wnt5a	164975	Person et al. [138]
Fuhrmann syndrome	228930	AR	Wnt7a	601570	Woods et al. [116]
Ulna and fibula, absence of, with severe limb deficiency	276820	AR	Wnt7a	601570	Woods et al. [116]
Odontoonychodermal dysplasia	257980	AR	Wnt10a	606268	Adaimy et al. [139]
Schopf-Schulz-Passarge syndrome	224750	AR	Wnt10a	606268	Bohring et al. [140]
Tooth agenesis, selective, 4	150400	AR, AD	Wnt10a	606268	Kantaputra and Sripathomsawat [111]
Split-hand/foot malformation 6	225300	AR	Wnt10b	601906	Ugur and Tolun [117]
Tooth agenesis, selective, 8	617073	AD	Wnt10b	601906	Yu et al. [112]
Receptor/coreceptor					
Robinow syndrome		AR	FZD2	600667	White et al. [141]
Nail disorder, nonsyndromic congenital, 10	614157	AR	FZD6	603409	Frojmark et al. [142]
Cenani-Lenz syndactyly syndrome	212780	AR	LRP4	604270	Li et al. [143]
Sclerosteosis 2	614305	AR, AD	LRP4	604270	Leupin et al. [132]
Osteopetrosis, autosomal dominant 1	607634	AD	LRP5	603506	Van Wesenbeeck et al. [122], Van Hul et al. [123]
Osteoporosis-pseudoglioma syndrome	259770	AR	LRP5	603506	Gong et al. [124]
Osteosclerosis	144750	AD	LRP5	603506	Van Wesenbeeck et al. [122]
Hyperostosis, endosteal	144750	AD	LRP5	603506	Van Wesenbeeck et al. [122]
Van Buchem disease, type 2	607636	AD	LRP5	603506	Van Wesenbeeck et al. [122], Little et al. [130]
Bone mineral density variability 1	601884	AD	LRP5	603506	Nguyen et al. [131]

Phenotype	Phenotype MIM number	Inheritance	Gene	Gene MIM number	Reference
Osteoporosis	166710	AD	LRP5	603506	Estrada et al. [121]
Tooth agenesis, selective, 7	616724	AD	LRP6	603507	Massink et al. [113]
Brachydactyly, type B1	113000	AD	ROR2	602337	Oldridge et al. [144]
Robinow syndrome, autosomal recessive	268310	AR	ROR2	602337	van Bokhoven et al. [145], Afzal et al. [146]
Simpson-Golabi-Behmel syndrome, type 1	312870	XLR	GPC3	300037	Pilia et al. [147]
Omodysplasia 1	258315	AR	GPC6	604404	Campos-Xavier et al. [148]
Fetal akinesia deformation sequence	208150	AR	MUSK	601296	Tan-Sindhunata et al. [149]
Antagonist					
Osteoarthritis susceptibility 1	165720	Mu	SFRP3	605083	Loughlin et al. [150]
Pyle disease	265900	AR	SFRP4	606570	Kiper et al. [129]
Craniodiaphyseal dysplasia, autosomal dominant	122860	AD	SOST	605740	Kim et al. [135]
Sclerosteosis 1	269500	AR	SOST	605740	Brunkow et al. [134]
Van Buchem disease	239100	AR	SOST	605740	Balemans et al. [133]
Agonists					
Robinow syndrome, autosomal dominant 2	616331	AD	DVL1	601365	White et al. [151]
Robinow syndrome, autosomal dominant 3	616894	AD	DVL3	601368	White et al. [152]
Bone mineral density, low, susceptibility to	615311		LGR4	606666	Styrkarsdottir et al. [128]
Palmoplantar hyperkeratosis with squamous cell carcinoma of skin and sex reversal	610644	AR	RSPO1	609595	Parma et al. [153]
Humerofemoral hypoplasia with radiotibial ray deficiency	618022		RSPO2	610575	Szenker-Ravi et al. [114]
Tetraamelia syndrome 2	618021		RSPO2	610575	Szenker-Ravi et al. [114]
Anonychia congenita	206800	AR	RSPO4	610573	Blaydon et al. [154]

Table 1.
Wnt signaling and human genetic bone diseases.

lists human genetic bone diseases caused by Wnt signaling disorders. Genotypic and phenotypic heterogeneity of genetic bone diseases–related Wnt signaling pathways is obvious. Tooth agenesis is caused by Wnt 10a, Wnt10b, and LRP6 by either autosomal dominant (AR) or autosomal recessive (AR) inheritance form [111–113]. Tetraamelia syndrome is skeletally characterized by limb agenesis or complete absence of limbs, bilateral cleft lip/palate, ankyloglossia, and mandibular hypoplasia with the pathogenic gene of Wnt3 and RSPO2 [114–115]. Other limb deficiency diseases in Wnt signaling includes Al-Awadi/Raas-Rothschild/Schinzel phocomelia syndrome (AARRS) (MIM 276820) and split-hand/foot malformation 6 (MIM 225300), with pathogenic gene of Wnt7a and Wnt10b, respectively [116, 117].

Robinow syndrome (RS) is characterized by facial features, orodental abnormalities, and hypoplastic genitalia [118]. All autosomal-dominant (DRS) and recessive (RRS) genes including Wnt5a, Dvl1, Dvl3, Fzd2, and ROR2 are involved in the Wnt/PCP pathways. This pathway plays an important role in the patterning and formation of the limb-bud outgrowth and growth plate in skeletal formation [119, 120].

Wnt signaling pathways are related to bone diseases with osteoporosis or high bone mass density (BMD) diseases. LRP5 gene is responsible for osteoporosis. Loss of function of LRP5 mutation causes osteoporosis (MIM 166710, 607634) and osteoporosis pseudoglioma syndrome (MIM 259770) [121–124]. Meanwhile, osteoporosis genes in Wnt signaling components include Wnt1, LGR4, and SFRP4. Wnt1 is the pathogenic gene for osteogenesis imperfect type XV (with bilateral mutations) and early onset osteoporosis (with heterozygous mutation) [125–127]. For LGR4, nonsense variation of c.376C-T is strongly associated with low bone mass density and osteoporotic fractures [128]. SFRP4 is the pathogenic gene for Pyle disease characterized by both osteoporosis and expanded trabecular metaphyses [129].

LRP5 is also the pathogenic gene for diseases with high BMD, Van Buchem syndrome type 2 (MIM 607636), bone mineral density variability (MIM 601884), osteosclerosis, and hyperostosis, endosteal (MIM 144750) [122, 130, 131]. LRP4 mutations lead to type I sclerosteosis (MIM 614305), which is also the disease with high BMD [132]. Sclerosteosis (SOST) gene mutation causes the high BMD diseases of Van Buchem syndrome (MIM 239100), sclerosteosis 1 (MIM 269500), and craniodiaphyseal dysplasia (MIM 122860) [133–135]. Sclerostin encoded by SOST gene is the endogenous Wnt signaling inhibitor, which interacts with LRP receptors [136]. Nowadays, monoclonal antibody of sclerostin is being tested in human clinical trials [137].

In all, the components of Wnt signaling including Wnt ligands, their receptors, coreceptors, antagonists, and agonists can cause different types of genetic bone diseases, which are related to both canonical and noncanonical Wnt signaling pathways. Study of Wnt signaling in genetic bone diseases and other human diseases provides promises for translational medicine.

5. Conclusions

We review the current status of Wnt signaling, including the secretion of Wnt ligands, and how Wnts binding to surface receptors trigger different intracellular response and transcription of different downstream target genes. However, the interactions among each components and the mechanisms of these interactions still need further study. Meanwhile, the cross talk network between canonical and noncanonical Wnt signaling, Wnt signaling, and other signaling pathways remains unsolved fully. Mutations in the components of Wnt signaling pathways lead to various genetic bone diseases and other genetic diseases. Genotypic and phenotypic heterozygosis is common in these genetic bone diseases. For the vital role of Wnt signaling components in bone diseases, potential drugs based on Wnt signaling is useful for treating different bone diseases.

Acknowledgements

The study was supported by the grants from the Shandong Provincial Natural Science Foundation of China (2015ZRC03171), Shandong Key Research and Development Plan (2016GSF201222).

Conflict of interest

No conflict of interest.

Author details

Yanqin Lu and Jinxiang Han
Shandong Academy of Medical Sciences, Jinan, China

*Address all correspondence to: yanqinlu@yahoo.com

References

[1] Nusse R, Varmus HE. Many tumors induced by the mouse mammary tumor virus contain a provirus integrated in the same region of the host genome. Cell. 1982;**31**:99-109

[2] Rijsewijk F, Schuermann M, Wagenaar E, Parren P, Weigel D, Nusse R. The Drosophila homolog of the mouse mammary oncogene int-1 is identical to the segment polarity gene wingless. Cell. 1987;**50**: 649-657

[3] McMahon AP, Moon RT. Ectopic expression of the proto-oncogene int-1 in Xenopus embryos leads to duplication of the embryonic axis. Cell. 1989;**58**:1075-1084

[4] Kusserow A, Pang K, Sturm C, Hrouda M, Lentfer J, Schmidt HA, et al. Unexpected complexity of the Wnt gene family in a sea anemone. Nature. 2005;**433**: 156-160

[5] Nusse R. An ancient cluster of Wnt paralogues. Trends in Genetics. 2001;**17**:443

[6] Shimizu H, Julius MA, Giarre M, Zheng Z, Brown AM, Kitajewski J. Transformation by Wnt family proteins correlates with regulation of beta-catenin. Cell Growth & Differentiation. 1997;**8**:1349-1358

[7] Janda CY, Waghray D, Levin AM, Thomas C, Garcia KC. Structural basis of Wnt recognition by Frizzled. Science. 2012;**337**:59-64

[8] Tanaka K, Kitagawa Y, Kadowaki T. Drosophila segment polarity gene product porcupine stimulates the posttranslational N-glycosylation of wingless in the endoplasmic reticulum. The Journal of Biological Chemistry. 2002;**277**:12816-12823

[9] Coudreuse D, Korswagen HC. The making of Wnt: New insights into Wnt maturation, sorting and secretion. Development. 2007;**134**:3-12

[10] Willert K, Brown JD, Danenberg E, Duncan AW, Weissman IL, Reya T, et al. Wnt proteins are lipid-modified and can act as stem cell growth factors. Nature. 2003; **423**:448-452

[11] Takada R, Satomi Y, Kurata T, Ueno N, Norioka S, Kondoh H, et al. Monounsaturated fatty acid modification of Wnt protein: Its role in Wnt secretion. Developmental Cell. 2006;**11**:791-801

[12] Franch-Marro X, Wendler F, Griffith J, Maurice MM, Vincent JP. In vivo role of lipid adducts on Wingless. Journal of Cell Science. 2008;**121**:1587-1592

[13] Ching W, Hang HC, Nusse R. Lipid-independent secretion of a Drosophila Wnt protein. The Journal of Biological Chemistry. 2008;**283**:17092-17098

[14] Parchure A, Vyas N, Mayor S. Wnt and Hedgehog: Secretion of lipid-modified morphogens. Trends in Cell Biology. 2018;**28**:157-170

[15] Rios-Esteves J, Haugen B, Resh MD. Identification of key residues and regions important for porcupine-mediated Wnt acylation. The Journal of Biological Chemistry. 2014;**289**:17009-17019

[16] Coombs GS, Yu J, Canning CA, Veltri CA, Covey TM, Cheong JK, et al. WLS-dependent secretion of WNT3A requires Ser209 acylation and vacuolar acidification. Journal of Cell Science. 2010;**123**: 3357-3367

[17] Herr P, Basler K. Porcupine-mediated lipidation is required for Wnt recognition by Wls. Developmental Biology. 2012;**361**:392-402

[18] Stabley JN, Towler DA. Arterial calcification in diabetes mellitus: Preclinical models and translational implications. Arteriosclerosis, Thrombosis, and Vascular Biology. 2017;**37**:205-217

[19] De Gregorio R, Pulcrano S, De Sanctis C, Volpicelli F, Guatteo E, von Oerthel L, et al. miR-34b/c regulates Wnt1 and enhances mesencephalic dopaminergic neuron differentiation. Stem Cell Reports. 2018;**10**: 1237-1250

[20] Gross JC, Zelarayan LC. The mingle-mangle of Wnt signaling and extracellular vesicles: Functional implications for heart research. Frontiers in Cardiovascular Medicine. 2018;**5**:10

[21] Peghaire C, Bats ML, Sewduth R, Jeanningros S, Jaspard B, Couffinhal T, et al. Fzd7 (Frizzled-7) expressed by endothelial cells controls blood vessel formation through Wnt/beta-catenin canonical signaling. Arteriosclerosis, Thrombosis, and Vascular Biology. 2016;**36**:2369-2380

[22] Komekado H, Yamamoto H, Chiba T, Kikuchi A. Glycosylation and palmitoylation of Wnt-3a are coupled to produce an active form of Wnt-3a. Genes to Cells. 2007;**12**:521-534

[23] Doubravska L, Krausova M, Gradl D, Vojtechova M, Tumova L, Lukas J, et al. Fatty acid modification of Wnt1 and Wnt3a at serine is prerequisite for lipidation at cysteine and is essential for Wnt signalling. Cellular Signalling. 2011;**23**: 837-848

[24] Tang X, Wu Y, Belenkaya TY, Huang Q, Ray L, Qu J, et al. Roles of N-glycosylation and lipidation in Wg secretion and signaling. Developmental Biology. 2012;**364**:32-41

[25] Kurayoshi M, Yamamoto H, Izumi S, Kikuchi A. Post-translational palmitoylation and glycosylation of Wnt-5a are necessary for its signalling. The Biochemical Journal. 2007;**402**:515-523

[26] Ching W, Nusse R. A dedicated Wnt secretion factor. Cell. 2006;**125**:432-433

[27] Nadanaka S, Kinouchi H, Kitagawa H. Histone deacetylase-mediated regulation of chondroitin 4-O-sulfotransferase-1 (Chst11) gene expression by Wnt/beta-catenin signaling. Biochemical and Biophysical Research Communications. 2016;**480**:234-240

[28] Kinoshita T, Maeda Y, Fujita M. Transport of glycosylphosphatidylinositol-anchored proteins from the endoplasmic reticulum. Biochimica et Biophysica Acta. 2013;**1833**: 2473-2478

[29] Das S, Yu S, Sakamori R, Stypulkowski E, Gao N. Wntless in Wnt secretion: Molecular, cellular and genetic aspects. Frontiers in Biology (Beijing). 2012;**7**:587-593

[30] Langton PF, Kakugawa S, Vincent JP. Making, exporting, and modulating Wnts. Trends in Cell Biology. 2016;**26**:756-765

[31] Banziger C, Soldini D, Schutt C, Zipperlen P, Hausmann G, Basler K. Wntless, a conserved membrane protein dedicated to the secretion of Wnt proteins from signaling cells. Cell. 2006;**125**:509-522

[32] Bartscherer K, Pelte N, Ingelfinger D, Boutros M. Secretion of Wnt ligands requires Evi, a conserved transmembrane protein. Cell. 2006;**125**:523-533

[33] Fu J, Jiang M, Mirando AJ, Yu HM, Hsu W. Reciprocal regulation of Wnt and Gpr177/mouse Wntless is required for embryonic axis formation. Proceedings of the National Academy of Sciences of the United States of America. 2009;**106**:18598-18603

[34] Zhong Z, Zylstra-Diegel CR, Schumacher CA, Baker JJ, Carpenter AC, Rao S, et al. Wntless functions in mature osteoblasts to regulate bone mass. Proceedings of the National Academy of Sciences of the United States of America. 2012;**109**:E2197-E2204

[35] Augustin I, Gross J, Baumann D, Korn C, Kerr G, Grigoryan T, et al. Loss of epidermal Evi/Wls results in a phenotype resembling psoriasiform dermatitis. The Journal of Experimental Medicine. 2013;**210**:1761-1777

[36] Cornett B, Snowball J, Varisco BM, Lang R, Whitsett J, Sinner D. Wntless is required for peripheral lung differentiation and pulmonary vascular development. Developmental Biology. 2013;**379**:38-52

[37] Yu J, Chia J, Canning CA, Jones CM, Bard FA, Virshup DM. WLS retrograde transport to the endoplasmic reticulum during Wnt secretion. Developmental Cell. 2014;**29**:277-291

[38] Buechling T, Chaudhary V, Spirohn K, Weiss M, Boutros M. p24 proteins are required for secretion of Wnt ligands. EMBO Reports. 2011;**12**:1265-1272

[39] Port F, Hausmann G, Basler K. A genome-wide RNA interference screen uncovers two p24 proteins as regulators of Wingless secretion. EMBO Reports. 2011;**12**:1144-1152

[40] Li X, Wu Y, Shen C, Belenkaya TY, Ray L, Lin X. Drosophila p24 and Sec22 regulate Wingless trafficking in the early secretory pathway. Biochemical and Biophysical Research Communications. 2015;**463**:483-489

[41] Panakova D, Sprong H, Marois E, Thiele C, Eaton S. Lipoprotein particles are required for Hedgehog and Wingless signalling. Nature. 2005;**435**:58-65

[42] Lorenowicz MJ, Korswagen HC. Sailing with the Wnt: Charting the Wnt processing and secretion route. Experimental Cell Research. 2009;**315**:2683-2689

[43] Port F, Kuster M, Herr P, Furger E, Banziger C, Hausmann G, et al. Wingless secretion promotes and requires retromer-dependent cycling of Wntless. Nature Cell Biology. 2008;**10**:178-185

[44] Yang PT, Lorenowicz MJ, Silhankova M, Coudreuse DY, Betist MC, Korswagen HC. Wnt signaling requires retromer-dependent recycling of MIG-14/Wntless in Wnt-producing cells. Developmental Cell. 2008;**14**:140-147

[45] Pan CL, Baum PD, Gu M, Jorgensen EM, Clark SG, Garriga G. *C. elegans* AP-2 and retromer control Wnt signaling by regulating mig-14/Wntless. Developmental Cell. 2008;**14**:132-139

[46] Hausmann G, Banziger C, Basler K. Helping Wingless take flight: How WNT proteins are secreted. Nature Reviews. Molecular Cell Biology. 2007;**8**:331-336

[47] Seaman MN. Recycle your receptors with retromer. Trends in Cell Biology. 2005;**15**:68-75

[48] Eaton S. Retromer retrieves wntless. Developmental Cell. 2008;**14**:4-6

[49] Yuasa T, Otani T, Koike T, Iwamoto M, Enomoto-Iwamoto M. Wnt/beta-catenin signaling stimulates matrix catabolic genes and activity in articular chondrocytes: Its possible role in joint degeneration. Laboratory Investigation. 2008;**88**:264-274

[50] Cullen PJ. Endosomal sorting and signalling: An emerging role for sorting nexins. Nature Reviews. Molecular Cell Biology. 2008;**9**:574-582

[51] Harterink M, Port F, Lorenowicz MJ, McGough IJ, Silhankova M, Betist MC, et al. A SNX3-dependent retromer pathway mediates retrograde transport of the Wnt sorting receptor Wntless and is required for Wnt secretion. Nature Cell Biology. 2011;**13**:914-923

[52] Johannes L, Wunder C. The SNXy flavours of endosomal sorting. Nature Cell Biology. 2011;**13**:884-886

[53] Zhang P, Zhou L, Pei C, Lin X, Yuan Z. Dysfunction of Wntless triggers the retrograde Golgi-to-ER transport of Wingless and induces ER stress. Scientific Reports. 2016;**6**:19418

[54] Ashe HL, Briscoe J. The interpretation of morphogen gradients. Development. 2006;**133**:385-394

[55] Korkut C, Ataman B, Ramachandran P, Ashley J, Barria R, Gherbesi N, et al. Trans-synaptic transmission of vesicular Wnt signals through Evi/Wntless. Cell. 2009;**139**:393-404

[56] Gross JC, Chaudhary V, Bartscherer K, Boutros M. Active Wnt proteins are secreted on exosomes. Nature Cell Biology. 2012;**14**:1036-1045

[57] Beckett K, Monier S, Palmer L, Alexandre C, Green H, Bonneil E, et al. Drosophila S2 cells secrete wingless on exosome-like vesicles but the wingless gradient forms independently of exosomes. Traffic. 2013;**14**:82-96

[58] Neumann S, Coudreuse DY, van der Westhuyzen DR, Eckhardt ER, Korswagen HC, Schmitz G, et al. Mammalian Wnt3a is released on lipoprotein particles. Traffic. 2009;**10**:334-343

[59] Bischoff M, Gradilla AC, Seijo I, Andres G, Rodriguez-Navas C, Gonzalez-Mendez L, et al. Cytonemes are required for the establishment of a normal Hedgehog morphogen gradient in Drosophila epithelia. Nature Cell Biology. 2013;**15**:1269-1281

[60] Stanganello E, Scholpp S. Role of cytonemes in Wnt transport. Journal of Cell Science. 2016;**129**:665-672

[61] Stanganello E, Hagemann AI, Mattes B, Sinner C, Meyen D, Weber S, et al. Filopodia-based Wnt transport during vertebrate tissue patterning. Nature Communications. 2015;**6**:5846

[62] Mulligan KA, Fuerer C, Ching W, Fish M, Willert K, Nusse R. Secreted Wingless-interacting molecule (Swim) promotes long-range signaling by maintaining Wingless solubility. Proceedings of the National Academy of Sciences of the United States of America. 2012;**109**:370-377

[63] Kimelman D, Xu W. Beta-catenin destruction complex: Insights and questions from a structural perspective. Oncogene. 2006;**25**:7482-7491

[64] Behrens J, Jerchow BA, Wurtele M, Grimm J, Asbrand C, Wirtz R, et al. Functional interaction of an axin homolog, conductin, with beta-catenin, APC, and GSK3beta. Science. 1998;**280**:596-599

[65] Yu N, Kakunda M, Pham V, Lill JR, Du P, Wongchenko M, et al. HSP105 recruits protein phosphatase 2A to dephosphorylate beta-catenin. Molecular and Cellular Biology. 2015;**35**:1390-1400

[66] Aberle H, Bauer A, Stappert J, Kispert A, Kemler R. Beta-catenin is a target for the ubiquitin-proteasome pathway. The EMBO Journal. 1997;**16**:3797-3804

[67] Bilic J, Huang YL, Davidson G, Zimmermann T, Cruciat CM, Bienz M, et al. Wnt induces LRP6 signalosomes and promotes dishevelled-dependent LRP6 phosphorylation. Science. 2007;**316**:1619-1622

[68] McGough IJ, Vincent JP. APC moonlights to prevent Wnt signalosome assembly. Developmental Cell. 2018;**44**:535-537

[69] Stadeli R, Hoffmans R, Basler K. Transcription under the control of nuclear Arm/beta-catenin. Current Biology. 2006;**16**:R378-R385

[70] Barker N, Clevers H. Mining the Wnt pathway for cancer therapeutics. Nature Reviews. Drug Discovery. 2006;**5**:997-1014

[71] Zeng X, Huang H, Tamai K, Zhang X, Harada Y, Yokota C, et al. Initiation of Wnt signaling: Control of Wnt coreceptor Lrp6 phosphorylation/activation via frizzled, dishevelled and axin functions. Development. 2008;**135**:367-375

[72] Tacchelly-Benites O, Wang Z, Yang E, Benchabane H. Axin phosphorylation in both Wnt-off and Wnt-on states requires the tumor suppressor APC. PLoS Genetics. 2018;**14**:e1007178

[73] Rubinfeld B, Albert I, Porfiri E, Fiol C, Munemitsu S, Polakis P. Binding of GSK3beta to the APC-beta-catenin complex and regulation of complex assembly. Science. 1996;**272**:1023-1026

[74] Neufeld KL, Zhang F, Cullen BR, White RL. APC-mediated downregulation of beta-catenin activity involves nuclear sequestration and nuclear export. EMBO Reports. 2000;**1**:519-523

[75] Sierra J, Yoshida T, Joazeiro CA, Jones KA. The APC tumor suppressor counteracts beta-catenin activation and H3K4 methylation at Wnt target genes. Genes & Development. 2006;**20**:586-600

[76] Aoki K, Taketo MM. Adenomatous polyposis coli (APC): A multi-functional tumor suppressor gene. Journal of Cell Science. 2007;**120**:3327-3335

[77] Takacs CM, Baird JR, Hughes EG, Kent SS, Benchabane H, Paik R, et al. Dual positive and negative regulation of wingless signaling by adenomatous polyposis coli. Science. 2008;**319**:333-336

[78] Su Y, Fu C, Ishikawa S, Stella A, Kojima M, Shitoh K, et al. APC is essential for targeting phosphorylated beta-catenin to the SCFbeta-TrCP ubiquitin ligase. Molecular Cell. 2008;**32**:652-661

[79] Saito-Diaz K, Benchabane H, Tiwari A, Tian A, Li B, Thompson JJ, et al. APC inhibits ligand-independent Wnt signaling by the clathrin endocytic pathway. Developmental Cell. 2018;**44**:566-581.e8

[80] Amit S, Hatzubai A, Birman Y, Andersen JS, Ben-Shushan E, Mann M, et al. Axin-mediated CKI phosphorylation of beta-catenin at Ser 45: A molecular switch for the Wnt pathway. Genes & Development. 2002;**16**:1066-1076

[81] Liu C, Li Y, Semenov M, Han C, Baeg GH, Tan Y, et al. Control of beta-catenin phosphorylation/degradation by a dual-kinase mechanism. Cell. 2002;**108**:837-847

[82] Wu G, Xu G, Schulman BA, Jeffrey PD, Harper JW, Pavletich NP. Structure of a beta-TrCP1-Skp1-beta-catenin complex: Destruction motif binding and lysine specificity of the SCF(beta-TrCP1) ubiquitin ligase. Molecular Cell. 2003;**11**:1445-1456

[83] Kitagawa M, Hatakeyama S, Shirane M, Matsumoto M, Ishida N, Hattori K, et al. An F-box protein, FWD1, mediates ubiquitin-dependent proteolysis of beta-catenin. The EMBO Journal. 1999;**18**:2401-2410

[84] Virshup DM, Shenolikar S. From promiscuity to precision: Protein phosphatases get a makeover. Molecular Cell. 2009;**33**:537-545

[85] Li X, Yost HJ, Virshup DM, Seeling JM. Protein phosphatase 2A and its B56 regulatory subunit inhibit Wnt signaling in Xenopus. The EMBO Journal. 2001;**20**:4122-4131

[86] Mitra A, Menezes ME, Pannell LK, Mulekar MS, Honkanen RE, Shevde LA, et al. DNAJB6 chaperones PP2A mediated dephosphorylation of GSK3beta to downregulate beta-catenin transcription target, osteopontin. Oncogene. 2012;**31**:4472-4483

[87] Seeling JM, Miller JR, Gil R, Moon RT, White R, Virshup DM. Regulation of beta-catenin signaling by the B56 subunit of protein phosphatase 2A. Science. 1999;**283**:2089-2091

[88] Eichhorn PJ, Creyghton MP, Bernards R. Protein phosphatase 2A regulatory subunits and cancer. Biochimica et Biophysica Acta. 2009;**1795**:1-15

[89] Yang J, Wu J, Tan C, Klein PS. PP2A:B56epsilon is required for Wnt/beta-catenin signaling during embryonic development. Development. 2003;**130**:5569-5578

[90] Yamamoto H, Hinoi T, Michiue T, Fukui A, Usui H, Janssens V, et al. Inhibition of the Wnt signaling pathway by the PR61 subunit of protein phosphatase 2A. The Journal of Biological Chemistry. 2001;**276**:26875-26882

[91] Zhang W, Yang J, Liu Y, Chen X, Yu T, Jia J, et al. PR55 alpha, a regulatory subunit of PP2A, specifically regulates PP2A-mediated beta-catenin dephosphorylation. The Journal of Biological Chemistry. 2009;**284**:22649-22656

[92] Hein AL, Seshacharyulu P, Rachagani S, Sheinin YM, Ouellette MM, Ponnusamy MP, et al. PR55alpha subunit of protein phosphatase 2A supports the tumorigenic and metastatic potential of pancreatic cancer cells by sustaining hyperactive oncogenic signaling. Cancer Research. 2016;**76**:2243-2253

[93] Strovel ET, Wu D, Sussman DJ. Protein phosphatase 2Calpha dephosphorylates axin and activates LEF-1-dependent transcription. The Journal of Biological Chemistry. 2000;**275**:2399-2403

[94] Vinyoles M, Del Valle-Perez B, Curto J, Padilla M, Villarroel A, Yang J, et al. Activation of CK1varepsilon by PP2A/PR61varepsilon is required for the initiation of Wnt signaling. Oncogene. 2017;**36**:429-438

[95] Schlessinger K, Hall A, Tolwinski N. Wnt signaling pathways meet Rho GTPases. Genes & Development. 2009;**23**:265-277

[96] Tepass U. The apical polarity protein network in Drosophila epithelial cells: Regulation of polarity, junctions, morphogenesis, cell growth, and survival. Annual Review of Cell and Developmental Biology. 2012;**28**:655-685

[97] Zallen JA. Planar polarity and tissue morphogenesis. Cell. 2007;**129**:1051-1063

[98] Casal J, Struhl G, Lawrence PA. Developmental compartments and planar polarity in Drosophila. Current Biology. 2002;**12**:1189-1198

[99] Zeidler MP, Perrimon N, Strutt DI. Multiple roles for four-jointed in planar polarity and limb patterning. Developmental Biology. 2000;**228**:181-196

[100] Simons M, Mlodzik M. Planar cell polarity signaling: From fly development to human disease. Annual Review of Genetics. 2008;**42**:517-540

[101] Strutt H, Gamage J, Strutt D. Robust asymmetric localization of planar polarity proteins is associated with organization into signalosome-like domains of variable stoichiometry. Cell Reports. 2016;**17**:2660-2671

[102] VanderVorst K, Hatakeyama J, Berg A, Lee H, Carraway III KL. Cellular and molecular mechanisms underlying planar cell polarity pathway contributions to cancer malignancy. Seminars in Cell & Developmental Biology. 2018;**81**:78-87

[103] Daulat AM, Borg JP. Wnt/planar cell polarity signaling: New opportunities for cancer treatment. Trends in Cancer. 2017;**3**:113-125

[104] Kuhl M, Sheldahl LC, Malbon CC, Moon RT. Ca(2+)/calmodulin-dependent protein kinase II is stimulated by Wnt and Frizzled homologs and promotes ventral cell fates in Xenopus. The Journal of Biological Chemistry. 2000;**275**:12701-12711

[105] Pereira C, Schaer DJ, Bachli EB, Kurrer MO, Schoedon G. Wnt5A/CaMKII signaling contributes to the inflammatory response of macrophages and is a target for the antiinflammatory action of activated protein C and interleukin-10. Arteriosclerosis, Thrombosis, and Vascular Biology. 2008;**28**:504-510

[106] Blumenthal A, Ehlers S, Lauber J, Buer J, Lange C, Goldmann T, et al. The Wingless homolog WNT5A and its receptor Frizzled-5 regulate inflammatory responses of human mononuclear cells induced by microbial stimulation. Blood. 2006;**108**:965-973

[107] Nishita M, Enomoto M, Yamagata K, Minami Y. Cell/tissue-tropic functions of Wnt5a signaling in normal and cancer cells. Trends in Cell Biology. 2010;**20**:346-354

[108] De A. Wnt/Ca2+ signaling pathway: A brief overview. Acta Biochimica et Biophysica Sinica. 2011;**43**:745-756

[109] Gong B, Shen W, Xiao W, Meng Y, Meng A, Jia S. The Sec14-like phosphatidylinositol transfer proteins Sec14l3/SEC14L2 act as GTPase proteins to mediate Wnt/Ca(2+) signaling. eLife 2017;**6**:e26362. DOI: 10.7554/eLife.26362

[110] Wang H, Lee Y, Malbon CC. PDE6 is an effector for the Wnt/Ca2+/cGMP-signalling pathway in development. Biochemical Society Transactions. 2004;**32**:792-796

[111] Kantaputra P, Sripathomsawat W. WNT10A and isolated hypodontia. American Journal of Medical Genetics. Part A. 2011;**155a**:1119-1122

[112] Yu P, Yang W, Han D, Wang X, Guo S, Li J, et al. Mutations in WNT10B are identified in individuals with oligodontia. American Journal of Human Genetics. 2016;**99**:195-201

[113] Massink MP, Creton MA, Spanevello F, Fennis WM, Cune MS, Savelberg SM, et al. Loss-of-function mutations in the WNT co-receptor LRP6 cause autosomal-dominant oligodontia. American Journal of Human Genetics. 2015;**97**:621-626

[114] Szenker-Ravi E, Altunoglu U, Leushacke M, Bosso-Lefevre C, Khatoo M, Thi Tran H, et al. RSPO2 inhibition of RNF43 and ZNRF3 governs limb development independently of LGR4/5/6. Nature. 2018;**557**:564-569

[115] Niemann S, Zhao C, Pascu F, Stahl U, Aulepp U, Niswander L, et al. Homozygous WNT3 mutation causes tetra-amelia in a large consanguineous family. American Journal of Human Genetics. 2004;**74**:558-563

[116] Woods CG, Stricker S, Seemann P, Stern R, Cox J, Sherridan E, et al. Mutations in WNT7A cause a range of limb malformations, including Fuhrmann syndrome and Al-Awadi/Raas-Rothschild/Schinzel phocomelia syndrome. American Journal of Human Genetics. 2006;**79**:402-408

[117] Ugur SA, Tolun A. Homozygous WNT10b mutation and complex inheritance in split-hand/foot malformation. Human Molecular Genetics. 2008;**17**:2644-2653

[118] Bain MD, Winter RM, Burn J. Robinow syndrome without mesomelic 'brachymelia': A report of five cases. Journal of Medical Genetics. 1986;**23**:350-354

[119] Li Y, Dudley AT. Noncanonical frizzled signaling regulates cell polarity of growth plate chondrocytes. Development. 2009;**136**:1083-1092

[120] Yamaguchi TP, Bradley A, McMahon AP, Jones S. A Wnt5a pathway underlies outgrowth of multiple structures in the vertebrate embryo. Development. 1999;**126**:1211-1223

[121] Estrada K, Styrkarsdottir U, Evangelou E, Hsu YH, Duncan EL, Ntzani EE, et al. Genome-wide meta-analysis identifies 56 bone mineral density loci and reveals 14 loci associated with risk of fractureNature Genetics. 2012;**44**:491-501

[122] Van Wesenbeeck L, Cleiren E, Gram J, Beals RK, Benichou O, Scopelliti D, et al. Six novel missense mutations in the LDL receptor-related protein 5 (LRP5) gene in different conditions with an increased bone density. American Journal of Human Genetics. 2003;**72**:763-771

[123] Van Hul E, Gram J, Bollerslev J, Van Wesenbeeck L, Mathysen D, Andersen PE, et al. Localization of the gene causing autosomal dominant osteopetrosis type I to chromosome 11q12-13. Journal of Bone and Mineral Research. 2002;**17**:1111-1117

[124] Gong Y, Slee RB, Fukai N, Rawadi G, Roman-Roman S, Reginato AM, et al. LDL receptor-related protein 5 (LRP5) affects bone accrual and eye development. Cell. 2001;**107**:513-523

[125] Pyott SM, Tran TT, Leistritz DF, Pepin MG, Mendelsohn NJ, Temme RT, et al. WNT1 mutations in families affected by moderately severe and progressive recessive osteogenesis imperfecta. American Journal of Human Genetics. 2013;**92**:590-597

[126] Keupp K, Beleggia F, Kayserili H, Barnes AM, Steiner M, Semler O, et al. Mutations in WNT1 cause different forms of bone fragility. American Journal of Human Genetics. 2013;**92**:565-574

[127] Laine CM, Joeng KS, Campeau PM, Kiviranta R, Tarkkonen K, Grover

M, et al. WNT1 mutations in early-onset osteoporosis and osteogenesis imperfecta. The New England Journal of Medicine. 2013;**368**:1809-1816

[128] Styrkarsdottir U, Thorleifsson G, Sulem P, Gudbjartsson DF, Sigurdsson A, Jonasdottir A, et al. Nonsense mutation in the LGR4 gene is associated with several human diseases and other traits. Nature. 2013;**497**:517-520

[129] Kiper POS, Saito H, Gori F, Unger S, Hesse E, Yamana K, et al. Cortical-bone fragility—Insights from sFRP4 deficiency in Pyle's disease. The New England Journal of Medicine. 2016;**374**:2553-2562

[130] Little RD, Carulli JP, Del Mastro RG, Dupuis J, Osborne M, Folz C, et al. A mutation in the LDL receptor-related protein 5 gene results in the autosomal dominant high-bone-mass trait. American Journal of Human Genetics. 2002;**70**:11-19

[131] Nguyen TV, Livshits G, Center JR, Yakovenko K, Eisman JA. Genetic determination of bone mineral density: Evidence for a major gene. The Journal of Clinical Endocrinology and Metabolism. 2003;**88**:3614-3620

[132] Leupin O, Piters E, Halleux C, Hu S, Kramer I, Morvan F, et al. Bone overgrowth-associated mutations in the LRP4 gene impair sclerostin facilitator function. The Journal of Biological Chemistry. 2011;**286**:19489-19500

[133] Balemans W, Patel N, Ebeling M, Van Hul E, Wuyts W, Lacza C, et al. Identification of a 52 kb deletion downstream of the SOST gene in patients with van Buchem disease. Journal of Medical Genetics. 2002;**39**:91-97

[134] Brunkow ME, Gardner JC, Van Ness J, Paeper BW, Kovacevich BR, Proll S, et al. Bone dysplasia sclerosteosis results from loss of the SOST gene product, a novel cystine knot-containing protein. American Journal of Human Genetics. 2001;**68**:577-589

[135] Kim SJ, Bieganski T, Sohn YB, Kozlowski K, Semenov M, Okamoto N, et al. Identification of signal peptide domain SOST mutations in autosomal dominant craniodiaphyseal dysplasia. Human Genetics. 2011;**129**:497-502

[136] Chang MK, Kramer I, Huber T, Kinzel B, Guth-Gundel S, Leupin O, et al. Disruption of Lrp4 function by genetic deletion or pharmacological blockade increases bone mass and serum sclerostin levels. Proceedings of the National Academy of Sciences of the United States of America. 2014;**111**:E5187-E5195

[137] Padhi D, Jang G, Stouch B, Fang L, Posvar E. Single-dose, placebo-controlled, randomized study of AMG 785, a sclerostin monoclonal antibody. Journal of Bone and Mineral Research. 2011;**26**:19-26

[138] Person AD, Beiraghi S, Sieben CM, Hermanson S, Neumann AN, Robu ME, et al. WNT5A mutations in patients with autosomal dominant Robinow syndrome. Developmental Dynamics. 2010;**239**:327-337

[139] Adaimy L, Chouery E, Megarbane H, Mroueh S, Delague V, Nicolas E, et al. Mutation in WNT10A is associated with an autosomal recessive ectodermal dysplasia: The odonto-onycho-dermal dysplasia. American Journal of Human Genetics. 2007;**81**:821-828

[140] Bohring A, Stamm T, Spaich C, Haase C, Spree K, Hehr U, et al. WNT10A mutations are a frequent cause of a broad spectrum of ectodermal dysplasias with sex-biased manifestation pattern in heterozygotes. American Journal of Human Genetics. 2009;**85**:97-105

[141] White JJ, Mazzeu JF, Coban-Akdemir Z, Bayram Y, Bahrambeigi V, Hoischen A, et al. WNT signaling perturbations underlie the genetic heterogeneity of Robinow syndrome. American Journal of Human Genetics. 2018;**102**:27-43

[142] Frojmark AS, Schuster J, Sobol M, Entesarian M, Kilander MBC, Gabrikova D, et al. Mutations in frizzled 6 cause isolated autosomal-recessive nail dysplasia. American Journal of Human Genetics. 2011;**88**:852-860

[143] Li Y, Pawlik B, Elcioglu N, Aglan M, Kayserili H, Yigit G, et al. LRP4 mutations alter Wnt/beta-catenin signaling and cause limb and kidney malformations in Cenani-Lenz syndrome. American Journal of Human Genetics. 2010;**86**:696-706

[144] Oldridge M, Fortuna AM, Maringa M, Propping P, Mansour S, Pollitt C, et al. Dominant mutations in ROR2, encoding an orphan receptor tyrosine kinase, cause brachydactyly type B. Nature Genetics. 2000;**24**:275-278

[145] van Bokhoven H, Celli J, Kayserili H, van Beusekom E, Balci S, Brussel W, et al. Mutation of the gene encoding the ROR2 tyrosine kinase causes autosomal recessive Robinow syndrome. Nature Genetics. 2000;**25**:423-426

[146] Afzal AR, Rajab A, Fenske CD, Oldridge M, Elanko N, Ternes-Pereira E, et al. Recessive Robinow syndrome, allelic to dominant brachydactyly type B, is caused by mutation of ROR2. Nature Genetics. 2000;**25**:419-422

[147] Pilia G, Hughes-Benzie RM, MacKenzie A, Baybayan P, Chen EY, Huber R, et al. Mutations in GPC3, a glypican gene, cause the Simpson-Golabi-Behmel overgrowth syndrome. Nature Genetics. 1996;**12**:241-247

[148] Campos-Xavier AB, Martinet D, Bateman J, Belluoccio D, Rowley L, Tan TY, et al. Mutations in the heparan-sulfate proteoglycan glypican 6 (GPC6) impair endochondral ossification and cause recessive omodysplasia. American Journal of Human Genetics. 2009;**84**:760-770

[149] Tan-Sindhunata MB, Mathijssen IB, Smit M, Baas F, de Vries JI, van der Voorn JP, et al. Identification of a Dutch founder mutation in MUSK causing fetal akinesia deformation sequence. European Journal of Human Genetics. 2015;**23**:1151-1157

[150] Loughlin J, Dowling B, Mustafa Z, Southam L, Chapman K. Refined linkage mapping of a hip osteoarthritis susceptibility locus on chromosome 2q. Rheumatology (Oxford). 2002;**41**:955-956

[151] White J, Mazzeu JF, Hoischen A, Jhangiani SN, Gambin T, Alcino MC, et al. DVL1 frameshift mutations clustering in the penultimate exon cause autosomal-dominant Robinow syndrome. American Journal of Human Genetics. 2015;**96**:612-622

[152] White JJ, Mazzeu JF, Hoischen A, Bayram Y, Withers M, Gezdirici A, et al. DVL3 alleles resulting in a −1 frameshift of the last exon mediate autosomal-dominant Robinow syndrome. American Journal of Human Genetics. 2016;**98**:553-561

[153] Parma P, Radi O, Vidal V, Chaboissier MC, Dellambra E, Valentini S, et al. R-spondin1 is essential in sex determination, skin differentiation and malignancy. Nature Genetics. 2006;**38**:1304-1309

[154] Blaydon DC, Ishii Y, O'Toole EA, Unsworth HC, Teh MT, Ruschendorf F, et al. The gene encoding R-spondin 4 (RSPO4), a secreted protein implicated in Wnt signaling, is mutated in inherited anonychia. Nature Genetics. 2006;**38**:1245-1247

Chapter 3

Potential Therapeutic Applications of Exosomes in Bone Regenerative Medicine

Jiazhao Yang, Wanbo Zhu, Jinsen Lu, Kai Xie, Shiyuan Fang and Lixin Kan

Abstract

The ability of bone regeneration is relatively robust, which is crucial for fracture healing, but delayed healing and nonunion are still common problems in clinical practice. Fortunately, exciting results have been achieved for regenerative medicine in recent years, especially in the area of stem cell-based treatment, but all these cell-based approaches face challenging problems, including immune rejection. For this reason, exosomes, stem cell-derived small vesicles of endocytic origin, have attracted the attention of many investigators in the field of bone regeneration. One of the attractive features of exosomes is that they are small and can travel between cells and deliver bioactive products, including miRNA, mRNA, proteins, and various other factors, to promote bone regeneration, with undetectable immune rejection. In this chapter, we intend to briefly update the recent progressions, and discuss the potential challenges in the target areas. Hopefully, our discussion would be helpful not only for the clinicians and the researchers in the specific disciplines but also for the general audiences as well.

Keywords: exosome, stem cell, fracture healing, osteogenesis, bone regeneration

1. Introduction

Fractures are common traumatic injuries during the entire human history. Both traditional and modern medicine have kept on exploring and researching on many potential treatments. Despite these efforts and relatively robust regenerative capacity of bone, currently, there are still about 5–10% fracture patients face delayed fracture healing and even nonunion, which has a great negative impact on the quality of life of patients as well as their families [1]. Surgical intervention with autologous bone graft seems to be the preferred method for such complication, but the secondary trauma and the limited resources of grafting bone make this approach still unsatisfactory [2, 3]. Other methods, including active substance injection and bone marrow transplantation, are also used clinically but they face their own challenges, including the effectiveness, safety and immune rejection [4, 5]. Therefore, how to promote fracture healing efficiently and safely is still the major focus of recent research in regenerative medicine for bone.

Normal bone regeneration is a complex but well-orchestrated physiological process that includes the initiation of ossification, osteoinduction, and osteogenesis

[6–9]. Specifically, when bone injury occurs, a series of signaling pathways is activated, which, in turn, leads to angiogenesis and other downstream events, and these together establish a favorable microenvironment, which set the stage for stem cell based fracture healing/regeneration [10]. Within this microenvironment, abundant blood vessels accelerate the metabolism while bringing a large number of multipotential stem cells [11, 12]. On the other hand, the mononuclear phagocyte system from the blood differentiates into osteoclasts in the newly established microenvironment, and the bone resorption, in turn, specifically stimulates the bone re-modeling process [13, 14]. During the stereotyped osteogenesis process, stem cells proliferate and differentiate into osteoblasts and migrate to areas of bone defects and bone resorption, secreting collagen matrices [7, 15–17], and then immature osteoblasts produce bone matrix containing calcium and phosphate to promote mineralization [18]. Of note, new blood vessels in the fracture microenvironment can also bring essential nutrients and mineral salt for fracture healing, improving the efficiency of osteogenic differentiation and bone regeneration [19].

Embryonic stem cell transplantation was considered as a potential promising treatment for tissue repair; however, due to the limitation of donor cells and biosafety issues, its clinical application has not been widely accepted [20–23]. Recently, it has been recognized that adult bone marrow-derived mesenchymal stem cells (BMSCs) might be a better alternative, and moreover, researchers found that BMSCs play an important role in promoting tissue regeneration through paracrine signaling [24, 25], in addition to directly differentiation into bony tissue. This paracrine effect, mediated by signaling molecules, transcription factors, and other proteins, regulates a series of signaling pathways involved in bone regeneration.

Interestingly, extracellular vesicle derived from stem cells under specific stimulation can carry specific substances produced by paracrine secretion and transmit to target organs/cells to act as an intercellular communicator [26, 27]. Among all the extracellular vesicles, the particles with the diameter around 40–100 nm are commonly called exosomes. Further study found, that in addition to stem cells, many other cells, such as osteoblasts, can also produce exosomes [28]. The key unanswered question is: could these different cell-derived exosomes promote bone regeneration and accelerate fracture healing? This chapter will focus on this important question.

2. A brief overview of exosome

In 1983, Harding found a lysosomal-like vesicle in reticulocytes of rats. It was found that transferrin was internalized by this vesicle and its receptors also recycled back to the plasma membrane through endocytosis [29]. In 1987, such vesicle-like structures were also found in the culture medium of sheep red blood cells cultured in vitro by Johnstone, and the vesicles were later named as exosomes [30]. It is now accepted that the extracellular vesicles secreted by cells could be generally classified as microvesicles, apoptotic bodies, and exosomes, on the basis of the size, cellular origin, content, and biological function [31, 32]. Currently, the exosomes are extensively studied. Exosomes, normally 40–100 nm in diameter, have been defined as a type of extracellular vesicles with unique biological features and morphology (flat or cup-shape under electron microscope) [33, 34] (**Figure 1**). The formation of exosome is essentially the encapsulation of bioactive substances, including proteins and nucleic acids, into multivesicular bodies with the help of endosomal sorting complex in the cells [35, 36]. The newly formed exosomes inside the cell are transported and fused with the plasma membrane and eventually released into the extracellular matrix [37, 38].

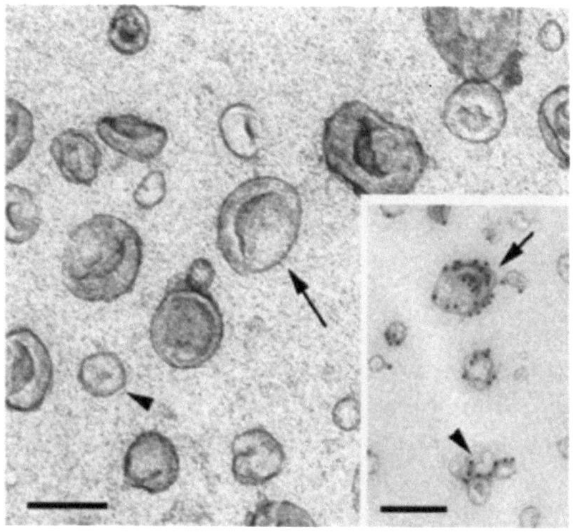

Figure 1.
Electron-microscopic observation of whole-mounted exosomes purified from mouse dendritic cells. Arrows indicate exosomes, arrowheads point to smaller nonexosomal vesicles. Scale bar = 100 nm. (Quote from Théry et al. [33].)

It is now known that numerous different type of cells, including dendritic cells, mast cells, lymphocytes, neurons, and endothelial cells secrete exosomes [39–43], which are found in blood, amniotic fluid, urine, malignant ascites, and other body fluids such as bile [44–47]. The key features of exosomes as intercellular communicators is due to the fact that they are able to selectively carry the contents of the parent cells and act on target cells [31, 38]. In 2007, Valadi found that exosomes contain RNA, which indicated exosomes might regulate genetic information flow [48]. In recent years, many studies have found that a variety of cell-derived exosomes contain mRNA and miRNA and play an important role in cell-to-cell signaling [48–50]. Therefore, the transport of RNA and active proteins through exosomes provides a novel pathway for activating target cell and initiating and propagating downstream signaling pathways. For example, in 2012, Cantaluppi discovered that microvesicles from epithelial progenitor-derived cell initiated renal-regeneration procedures by carrying miRNAs and acting on target cells, reversing focal ischemic lesions [51].

The regenerative effects of exosomes have been validated in other tissues and organs, including the heart, lungs, kidneys, and brain [52–54]. For example, in a mouse model of myocardial infarction, treatment of exosomes can improve cardiac epicardial remodeling and increase left ventricular ejection fraction [55]. In hypoxic-induced pulmonary hypertension, exosome treatment inhibits disease progression and protects the lungs from hypertension [56]. In addition, exosome treatment can improve renal function in a mouse model of acute kidney injury [57]. These studies indicate that exosomes have the capacity to promote tissue regeneration, which provides a basis for their potential application in bone regeneration [58].

3. Exosomes in bone regeneration

3.1 The exosomes derived from different cells promote bone regeneration

The mechanism of stem cells in the treatment of diseases has not been fully elucidated; however, it is now commonly accepted that there are two recognized mechanisms: differentiation and paracrine. In fact, it is becoming clearer that paracrine mechanism could be a more important mechanism; therefore, exosomes, as important mediators in paracrine mechanism, have attracted researchers.

Embryonic stem cells are considered to be the ideal materials for regenerative medicine because of their ability of pluripotent differentiation. But later study found that bone marrow mesenchymal stem cell (BMSC) could be a better alternative, i.e., BMSCs are self-renewing mesodermal pluripotent stem cells that can differentiate into osteoblasts, fat cells, nerve cells, and myoblasts [24, 59]. Recent study also found that BMSCs' roles in inducing angiogenesis, regulating inflammation, inhibiting apoptosis, and regulating osteogenesis differentiation make them desirable for bone regeneration applications [59].

Similarly, the adipose-derived stem cells (ADSCs) can also be osteogenic differentiated to promote bone regeneration, when they have been applied to the bone defects using a composite biological scaffold [60]. In addition, endothelial progenitor cells (EPCs) can differentiate into vascular endothelial cells to generate blood vessels, and promote MSCs osteogenesis in a specific microenvironment [61, 62]. Also, differentiated cells, such as osteoblasts and osteoclasts, also have the ability to promote bone regeneration [15, 26].

More importantly, numerous studies suggest that the above-mentioned cell-derived exosomes all have a certain ability to promote bone regeneration, through regulating bone regeneration procedures such as angiogenesis, osteogenic differentiation, and bone mineral deposition. However, the capacities and regeneration mechanisms of exosomes from different derived cells are somewhat inconsistent, likely due to their different contents.

3.2 Genetic materials carried by exosomes regulate bone regeneration

It was reported that stem cell-derived exosomes can carry genetic materials such as miRNA and mRNA, and share these genetic information between mature bone cells and stem/progenitor cells, which is an important way to promote bone regeneration [63]. MicroRNAs (miRNAs) are thought to be important posttranscriptional regulators of osteoblast-associated osteogenesis and bone remodeling, enabling a range of bone regenerative responses [64, 65]. Interestingly, miRNAs, inside the lipid membrane of exosomes, can avoid the decomposition of immune system; therefore, they exert their effects more efficiently [66].

Many researchers reported that some stem cell-derived exosomal miRNAs have the ability to activate osteogenic differentiation and angiogenesis of target cells and promote bone formation. For example, Xu first found that exosomal miRNA is a regulator of osteoblast differentiation [67]. Similarly, a series of miRNAs, such as let-7a, which could enhance the osteogenic differentiation of stem cells and promote bone regeneration, are significantly upregulated [68]. These data all demonstrated that stem cell-derived exosomes could promote bone regeneration by carrying specific miRNAs (**Table 1**).

Furthermore, many recent studies focus on MSCs-derived exosomes (BMSC-Exo) for bone regeneration. For examples, in CD9−/− mice, BMSC-Exo isolated from culture medium can accelerate fracture healing compared with the control group [69]. In vitro analysis of the exosomes revealed that miR-21, miR-4332 and other osteogenic differentiation-related miRNAs are highly expressed compared to other cell-derived exosomes. Interestingly, mononuclear cell chemotactic protein MCP-1/-3 and stromal cell-derived factor SDF-1, were lower in BMSC-Exo than in the control group [70, 71]. This might suggest that differential distribution of osteogenic differentiation and angiogenesis-related miRNAs in BMSC-Exo. In another study, BMSC-Exo group showed a significant increase in bone formation and repair rate in the model of mouse skull repair, compared with the control group. Similarly, in vitro experiments,

miRNA	Derived cells	Express level	Target cells	In vivo evaluation	In vitro evaluation	Involved pathway
Let-7a [67]	BMSCs	Upregulated	MSCs	Promote bone formation	Promote osteogenesis and suppress adipogenesis [68]	AXIN2 HMGA2
miR-218 [67]	BMSCs	Upregulated	SMSCs	None	Inhibit osteogenic differentiation	None
miR-203 [67]	BMSCs	Upregulated	BMSCs	None	Promote osteoblastic differentiation	None
miR-196a [59]	BMSCs	Upregulated	BMSCs	Stimulate bone formation	Positively regulated osteogenic genes and osteoblastic differentiation but did not inhibit proliferation	None
miR-27a [59]	BMSCs	Upregulated	MSCs	Overexpression promoted osteogenic differentiation	None	PPARγ
miR-206 [59]	BMSCs	Upregulated	None	None	None	None
miR-21 [69]	BMSCs	Upregulated	BMSCs/ MSCs	Accelerate fracture healing	Promote osteogenic differentiation	PI3K/AKT
miR-125b [69]	BMSCs	Upregulated	BMSCs	None	Suppresses the proliferation and osteogenic differentiation of BMSCs	None
miR-10b [72]	BMSCs	Upregulated	MSCs	None	Promote the migration of MSCs	None
miR-221 [72]	BMSCs/ MSCs	Downregulated	MSCs	Anti-miR-221 enhances bone healing	Downregulation of miR-221 triggers osteogenic differentiation	None
miR-155 [67]	BMSCs	Downregulated	None	None	None	None
miR-31 [72]	MSCs	Downregulated	BMSCs	Inhibition of miR-31 in MSCs increased bone volume and bone mineral density	Inhibit the osteogenic differentiation of MSCs	Wnt
miR-144 [72]	MSCs	Downregulated	MSCs	None	Inhibit the osteogenic differentiation of MSCs	None

Table 1.
Summary of Exosomal miRNAs and their potential effects on bone metabolism.

BMSC-Exo was showed to activate osteogenic differentiation, increase osteoblast activity, and promote bone formation without inhibiting stem cell proliferation [59].

Further study found that the ability of exosomes to promote bone formation is different even when the parent cells are in different differentiation stages. For example, in vitro experiments demonstrated that the human mesenchymal stem cell-derived exosomes (hMSCs-Exo) from the late differential stage have the strongest osteogenic differentiation ability [67, 72]. Consistently, MiR-31, miR-221, and miR-144 that inhibit osteogenic differentiation have significant decreased levels in late differential stage of hMSCs-Exo, while miR-21, miR-10b, and other miRNAs that contribute to osteogenesis is significantly upregulated [73–76]. It should be noted that the exosome miRNA's ability to regulate cell function could be context dependent, especially in the present of inhibitory miRNAs [67, 77]. Therefore, to promote bone regeneration using stem cell-derived exosomes, silencing inhibitory miRNAs may be a problem to be solved.

In addition, some miRNAs carried by other cell-derived exosomes also have the ability to promote bone regeneration. For example, the mineralization-related miR-503-3p is highly expressed in the miRNAs carried by osteoblast-derived exosomes. Interestingly, miR-503-3p also inhibits osteoclast differentiation by mediating RANK expression [78]. Osteoblast-derived exosomes and pre-osteoblasts-derived cells can also carry miRNAs such as let-7a and miR-96a, which have been previously confirmed to be involved in bone remodeling [79]. Similarly, the miR-27a-3p carried by myogenic cell-derived exosomes can also enhance osteogenic differentiation of pre-osteoblasts [80]. In contrast, osteoclast-derived exosomes can carry miRNAs such as miR-214 that inhibit osteogenic differentiation of osteoblasts [81]. Interestingly, in vitro experiments have found that human adipose stem cell-derived exosomes (ASCs-Exo) can increase the osteogenic capacity of target cells by upregulating the mRNA expression of osteogenesis-related genes RUNX2, ALP, and COL1A1, and promote bone formation [82]. In addition, the mRNA of RAB13, an osteoclastic membrane trafficking protein required for bone resorption, is also overrepresented in osteoblast-derived exosome [49].

Overall, cell-derived exosomal miRNAs and mRNAs likely play important roles in bone regeneration, through promoting osteogenic differentiation, angiogenesis and other processes. However, it is unclear whether protein factors are eventually needed to mediate their final effects.

3.3 Key protein factors carried by exosomes regulate bone regeneration

Key factors in stem cell-derived exosomes are known to mediate a series of conserved signaling pathways.

RUNX2 is an important transcription factor that can regulate osteogenesis differentiation, through promoting the differentiation of pluripotent stem cells into osteoblasts and inhibit osteoblast maturation [83]. Consistently, in vivo experiment found that human induced pluripotent mesenchymal stem cell-derived exosomes (hiPS-MSC-Exo) stimulated osteogenic differentiation, promoted angiogenesis, and improved fracture healing rate in animals with the upregulated transcription factors such as RUNX2 [84]. It was also reported that cell derived exosomal miRNAs are critical for upregulation of RUNX2 [85, 86]. Interestingly, RUNX2 directly represses miR-31 expression, which significantly inhibits expression of the osteogenic transcription factors OPN, BSP, Osterix (OSX), and OCN [87].

PI3K-AKT signaling pathway is thought to play an important role in exosomes-mediated bone regeneration because it stimulates osteogenic differentiation and promotes osteogenesis [88, 89]. Consistently, Shabbir et al. found that BMSCs-Exo activates multiple signaling pathways including Akt, Erk1/2, and STAT3 to induce angiogenic responses in fibroblasts [90]. In vitro experiment also found that hiPS-MSC-Exo downregulates inhibitory factor (GSK3β and PTEN) by upregulating PI3K-AKT target genes PDGFA and FGFR1 [91], and activation of PI3K-AKT cascade induces stem cell proliferation and differentiation into osteoblasts, and enhances ALP expression and calcium salt deposition, promoting bone regeneration. In the context of long-term nonunion of the femoral neck fracture or intertrochanteric fracture induces femoral head necrosis, Liu et al. found that iPS-MSCs-Exo activates the PI3K/Akt signaling pathway to increase angiogenesis and reduce bone loss [94].

miRNAs are also important molecules that regulate the PI3K-AKT signaling pathway. For example, miR-21, highly expressed in BMSCs-Exo, is one of the major regulators in stem cell-derived exosomes, which promotes osteogenic differentiation not only by inhibiting SOX2 [92], but also regulating the PI3K-AKT-GSK3β signaling pathway, which, in turn, activates the transcription of RUNX2, and stimulate osteogenic differentiation [93].

Wnt pathway is an important signaling pathway related to bone repair. In this regard, ASCs-Exo pretreated with TNF-α could upregulate Wnt3 expression in stem cells and promote bone regeneration [95, 96]. Zhang et al. also found that human umbilical cord stem cell-derived exosomes induce Wnt4-mediated β-catenin nuclear transport, and induce endothelial cell proliferation, differentiation, and neovascularization [97]. Similarly, BMSCs-Exo also activates the Wnt3a-β-catenin pathway and induces angiogenic capacity of fibroblast [98].

RANKL-RANK signaling is known to be responsible for homeostasis of bone metabolism, which is determined by a dynamic balance between osteoclasts and osteoblast [99]. Interestingly, Nuclear factor kappaB ligand (RANKL) can be encapsulated into osteoblast exosomes, while osteoclast exosomes are enriched with RANK [100]. When RANKL binds to RANK in pre-osteoclasts, TNF receptor-related factors (TRAF) 2, 3, 5, and 6 are recruited, leading to activation of multiple signaling pathways including MAPK and NF-κB, promoting osteoclast differentiation and bone resorption [101]. Moreover, level of RANK-containing exosomes increases in the late stage of osteoclast differentiation, which negatively feedbacks on RANKL-RANK signaling to inhibit osteoclast differentiation [99]. Therefore, RANKL-RANK loop contributes to the homeostasis of bone metabolism and bone regeneration.

Other proteins and cytokines in the exosomes are also involved in promoting bone regeneration process. For example, Martins et al. found that hBMSCs-Exo induced BMP2 upregulation, and BMP2 in turn, promoted stem cell osteogenic differentiation and osteogenesis by cascade activation of transcription factor OSX instead of RUNX2 [65]. Similarly, SPE1 (secreted phosphoprotein 1), integrin-binding sialoprotein and bone gland protein BGLAP (bone g-carboxyglutamate (gla) protein) were also upregulated, which facilitated bone mineralization and other bone regeneration processes. MSCs-Exo is also known to induce high expression of BMP9, transforming growth factor β1 (TGFβ1), vascular endothelial growth factor (VEGF), and platelet-derived growth factor (PDGF) [102]. BMP9 is considered to be an osteogenic factor stronger than BMP2. TGFβ1 and PDGF are known to play roles both in osteogenic differentiation and angiogenesis [103–105]. Qi et al. also found that hiPSC-MSC-Exo induced high expression of osteopontin, osteocalcin, and type I collagen (COL1), and enhanced bone mineralization [84, 106]. Meanwhile, high expression of phosphorylated protein and bone matrix acidic protein (DMP1) was found in the extracellular matrix (ECM) containing MSCs-Exo, suggesting MSCs-Exo promotes calcium phosphate recruitment and bone mineralization [107].

In addition, exosomes from osteoblast carry transforming growth factor beta receptor II interacting protein1 (TRIP-1), a regulator of osteoblast function. TRIP-1 from the exosomes can bind to type I collagen and promote its mineralized extracellular matrix, therefore bone mineralizing [108]. Sema4D is an osteoclast membrane protein that can be carried in exosomes derived from osteoclasts and acts on the receptor Plexin B on osteoblasts [81]. The Sema4D-Plexin B interaction promotes the release the content of exosomes and accelerates bone formation.

It is worthy to mention that some proteins, though are highly expressed in stem cell-derived exosomes and have the potential for bone regeneration, do not seem to play important roles in exosomes mediated osteogenic or chondrogenic differentiation in different contexts. For example, heat-shock protein 70 (HSP70), which can be used as a marker of BMSCs-Exo, is downregulated in human MSC-Exos and negatively affects osteogenic and chondrogenic differentiation. Similarly, down-regulation of heat shock protein B8 (HSPB8) can reduce the formation of dental pulp stem cells, and osteogenic differentiation ability [109-111]. Overall, the specific biological mechanisms of some functional proteins to promote fracture healing are not fully understood, and further detailed researches will be needed.

4. Clinical therapeutic applications and limitations

Many studies have shown that stem-derived exosomes in vitro and in vivo activate a series of bone regeneration programs through their selective bioactive substances, which are mainly through osteogenic differentiation, angiogenesis, and bone mineralization. In these applications, the high extracellular matrix binding affinity of stem cell-derived exosomes is a big plus for their clinical application. Recently, some scholars have found that human adipose-derived stem cell-derived exosomes promote fracture healing in animals by binding to polylactic acid-glycolic acid scaffolds [82]. At the same time, the immunomodulatory and anti-inflammatory properties of stem cell-derived exosomes have also attracted the attention of researchers, which could be the potential biological mechanisms for clinical treatment to promote bone regeneration [112, 113].

However, so far there are few examples of clinical trials using exosomes as clinical treatments. At present, exosome clinical application has only been reported in the fields of treatment of chronic kidney disease, type 1 diabetes mellitus (clinical trialNCT02138331), and skin damage (clinical trial NCT02565264) [114]. In the field of bone regeneration, to our best knowledge, there is not any clinical trial, either ongoing or finished. The main reasons for this delay could be logistic, since the separation, acquisition, purification, and identification of exosomes are still in the laboratory stage, and large scale manufacture is still a major practical challenge. In addition, the healing of the fracture will take several months, and how to make the exosomes available constantly in the fracture site for such a long time is also a problem.

Cell culture: The acquisition of a large number of exosomes requires a large number of cells [115]. However, large scale stem cells culture may alter the cell phenotype [116]. Existing cell culture techniques such as bioreactors have expanded the surface area of cell growth, but it is still difficult to perfectly control the conditions of cell growth [117]. As mentioned above, exosomes from different stages of derived cells have different bone regeneration capabilities. However, there are still limitations on how to obtain batch production from the specific stage of the cells.

Purification: Ultracentrifugation and ultrafiltration can be used to obtain purified exosomes in the laboratory, but this technology is difficult to apply on a large scale [118]. The nonspecific precipitation method using polyethyleneglycol (PEG) can solve this problem well, but PEG needs to be removed again in the product, which is technical challenging [119]. The tangential-flow filtration technology based on cell size separation is currently considered promising; however, it is expensive to use and does not separate some biological materials such as DNA [118, 120].

Identification and quality control: Current laboratory identification and quality control methods include direct observation under electron microscopy and biomarkers observation, but none of them can be scaled up easily. The identification and quality control using immunomagnetic capture of exosomal biomarkers through microfluidic technology can speed up the identification process, but it also has a long way to go before this method can be commonly accepted [118, 121].

In summary, the existing technology still has great challenges for large-scale acquisition of purified exosomes.

5. Existing disputes and problems

Whether promoting bone regeneration will indirectly lead to tumor production is a controversy that needs to be tested seriously. In fact, there are some studies have shown that exosomes can promote tumor growth and malignant transformation or inhibit tumor survival [122, 123]. For example, Qi et al. found that BMSCs-Exo can induce osteosarcoma growth by activating the Hedgehog signaling pathway [124]. BMSCs-Exo can induce drug resistance even on the basis of promoting the proliferation and differentiation of myeloma cells and the survival of migration [125, 126]. How to limit the potential tumor-promoting ability of stem cell-derived exosomes is a problem that must be solved before clinical application. However, miR-340 carried by early BMSCs-Exo can inhibit the angiogenic ability of myeloma thus significantly limiting tumor growth [127].

In clinical applications, while the short term activity of pro-osteogenic differentiation in vitro or promotion of bone regeneration is observed by exosomes treatment, the long-term activity that affects the quality of fracture healing or osteophyte formation is unknown. It is also unclear how to stop the biological effects of exosomes when the satisfactory therapeutic effect is achieved. To clarify these issues, at present, it is urgently needed to test exosomes in animal model before we can move on to clinical study.

6. Conclusion

In summary, exosomes with their carried bioactive contents have a capacity to promote bone regeneration through osteogenic differentiation, angiogenesis, and bone mineralization (**Figure 2**). Hence, exosomes are identified as potential

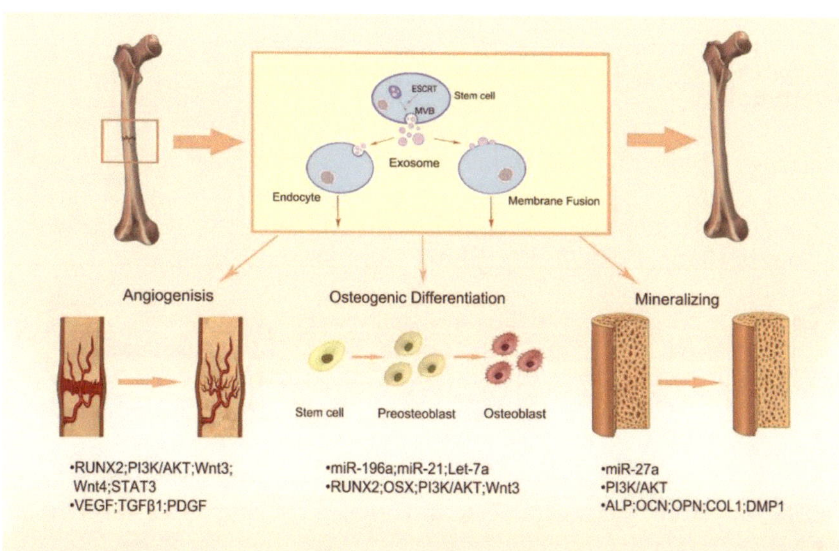

Figure 2.
Main biological mechanism of therapeutic application exosomes in bone regenerative medicine.

new "acellular" therapeutic application in bone regenerative medicine. However, clinical application of exosomes still faces controversies and challenges, and further researches are needed to elucidate the signaling pathway, molecular mechanism, and long-term clinical effect.

Acknowledgements

We appreciate the help from many members of the Kessler Lab. LK was supported in part by national natural science foundation of China (81472087) and natural science foundation of Anhui province (1508085MC45).

Conflict of interest

The authors declare no competing interests.

Author details

Jiazhao Yang[1], Wanbo Zhu[1], Jinsen Lu[1], Kai Xie[1], Shiyuan Fang[1] and Lixin Kan[2*]

1 Department of Orthopedics, The First Hospital of University of Science and Technology of China, Hefei, Anhui, China

2 Department of Neurology, Northwestern University, Chicago, USA

*Address all correspondence to: l-kan@northwestern.edu

References

[1] Huang W, Zhang K, Zhu Y, Wang Z, Li Z, Zhang J. Genetic polymorphisms of NOS2 and predisposition to fracture non-union: A case control study based on Han Chinese population. PLoS One. 2018;**13**:e193673. DOI: 10.1371/journal.pone.0193673

[2] Ehrler DM, Vaccaro AR. The use of allograft bone in lumbar spine surgery. Clinical Orthopaedics and Related Research. 2000:38-45

[3] Stafford PR, Norris BL. Reamer-irrigator-aspirator bone graft and bi Masquelet technique for segmental bone defect nonunions: A review of 25 cases. Injury. 2010;**41**:S72-S77. DOI: 10.1016/S0020-1383(10)70014-0

[4] Hernigou P, Poignard A, Beaujean F, Rouard H. Percutaneous autologous bone-marrow grafting for nonunions. Influence of the number and concentration of progenitor cells. The Journal of Bone and Joint Surgery. American Volume. 2005;**87**:1430-1437. DOI: 10.2106/JBJS.D.02215

[5] Kawaguchi H, Oka H, Jingushi S, Izumi T, Fukunaga M, Sato K, et al. A local application of recombinant human fibroblast growth factor 2 for tibial shaft fractures: A randomized, placebo-controlled trial. Journal of Bone and Mineral Research. 2010;**25**:2735-2743. DOI: 10.1002/jbmr.146

[6] Cornell CN, Lane JM. Current understanding of osteoconduction in bone regeneration. Clinical Orthopaedics and Related Research. 1998;**Res**:S267-S273. PMID: 9917646

[7] Javed A, Chen H, Ghori FY. Genetic and transcriptional control of bone formation. Oral and Maxillofacial Surgery Clinics of North America. 2010;**22**:283-293. DOI: 10.1016/j.coms.2010.05.001

[8] Salgado CL, Grenho L, Fernandes MH, Colaco BJ, Monteiro FJ. Biodegradation, biocompatibility, and osteoconduction evaluation of collagen-nanohydroxyapatite cryogels for bone tissue regeneration. Journal of Biomedical Materials Research. Part A. 2016;**104**:57-70. DOI: 10.1002/jbm.a.35540

[9] Albrektsson T, Johansson C. Osteoinduction, osteoconduction and osseointegration. European Spine Journal. 2001;**10**(Suppl 2):S96-S101. DOI: 10.1007/s005860100282

[10] Percival CJ, Richtsmeier JT. Angiogenesis and intramembranous osteogenesis. Developmental Dynamics. 2013;**242**:909-922. DOI: 10.1002/dvdy.23992

[11] Stegen S, van Gastel N, Carmeliet G. Bringing new life to damaged bone: The importance of angiogenesis in bone repair and regeneration. Bone. 2015;**70**:19-27. DOI: 10.1016/j.bone.2014.09.017

[12] Ando Y, Matsubara K, Ishikawa J, Fujio M, Shohara R, Hibi H, et al. Stem cell-conditioned medium accelerates distraction osteogenesis through multiple regenerative mechanisms. Bone. 2014;**61**:82-90. DOI: 10.1016/j.bone.2013.12.029

[13] Chambers TJ. The birth of the osteoclast. Annals of the New York Academy of Sciences. 2010;**1192**:19-26. DOI: 10.1111/j.1749-6632.2009.05224.x

[14] Boyce BF. Advances in the regulation of osteoclasts and osteoclast functions. Journal of Dental Research. 2013;**92**:860-867. DOI: 10.1177/0022034513500306

[15] Matsuo K, Irie N. Osteoclast–osteoblast communication. Archives of Biochemistry and Biophysics.

2008;**473**:201-209. DOI: 10.1016/j.abb.2008.03.027

[16] Komori T. Regulation of osteoblast differentiation by transcription factors. Journal of Cellular Biochemistry. 2006;**99**:1233-1239. DOI: 10.1002/jcb.20958

[17] Capulli M, Paone R, Rucci N. Osteoblast and osteocyte: Games without frontiers. Archives of Biochemistry and Biophysics. 2014;**561**:3-12. DOI: 10.1016/j.abb.2014.05.003

[18] Dirckx N, Van Hul M, Maes C. Osteoblast recruitment to sites of bone formation in skeletal development, homeostasis, and regeneration. Birth Defects Research Part C: Embryo Today: Reviews. 2013;**99**:170-191. DOI: 10.1002/bdrc.21047

[19] Saran U, Gemini Piperni S, Chatterjee S. Role of angiogenesis in bone repair. Archives of Biochemistry and Biophysics. 2014;**561**:109-117. DOI: 10.1016/j.abb.2014.07.006

[20] Katsara O, Mahaira LG, Iliopoulou EG, Moustaki A, Antsaklis A, Loutradis D, et al. Effects of donor age, gender, and In vitro cellular aging on the phenotypic, functional, and molecular characteristics of mouse bone marrow-derived mesenchymal stem cells. Stem Cells and Development. 2011;**20**:1549-1561. DOI: 10.1089/scd.2010.0280

[21] Hass R, Kasper C, Bohm S, Jacobs R. Different populations and sources of human mesenchymal stem cells (MSC): A comparison of adult and neonatal tissue-derived MSC. Cell Communication and Signaling: CCS. 2011;**9**:12. DOI: 10.1186/1478-811X-9-12

[22] Bléry P, Corre P, Malard O, Sourice S, Pilet P, Amouriq Y, et al. Evaluation of new bone formation in irradiated areas using association of mesenchymal stem cells and total fresh bone marrow mixed with calcium phosphate scaffold. Journal of Materials Science: Materials in Medicine. 2014;**25**:2711-2720. DOI: 10.1007/s10856-014-5282-5

[23] Hao Z, Wang S, Zhang X, Lu J. Stem cell therapy: A promising biological strategy for tendon-bone healing after anterior cruciate ligament reconstruction. Cell Proliferation. 2016;**49**:154-162. DOI: 10.1111/cpr.12242

[24] Burdon TJ, Paul A, Noiseux N, Prakash S, Shum-Tim D. Bone marrow stem cell derived paracrine factors for regenerative medicine: Current perspectives and therapeutic potential. Bone Marrow Research. 2011;**2011**:1-14. DOI: 10.1155/2011/207326

[25] Sharma RI, Snedeker JG. Paracrine interactions between mesenchymal stem cells affect substrate driven differentiation toward tendon and bone phenotypes. PLoS One. 2012;**7**:e31504. DOI: 10.1371/journal.pone.0031504

[26] Liu M, Sun Y, Zhang Q. Emerging role of extracellular vesicles in bone remodeling. Journal of Dental Research. 2018;**97**(8):859-868. DOI: 10.1177/0022034518764411

[27] Keshtkar S, Azarpira N, Ghahremani MH. Mesenchymal stem cell-derived extracellular vesicles: Novel frontiers in regenerative medicine. Stem Cell Research & Therapy. 2018;**9**(1):63. DOI: 10.1186/s13287-018-0791-7

[28] Golchin A, Hosseinzadeh S, Ardeshirylajimi A. The exosomes released from different cell types and their effects in wound healing. Journal of Cellular Biochemistry. 2018;**119**(7):5043-5052. DOI: 10.1002/jcb.26706

[29] Harding C, Heuser J, Stahl P. Receptor-mediated endocytosis of transferrin and recycling of the transferrin receptor in rat reticulocytes. The Journal of Cell Biology. 1983;**97**:329-339

[30] Johnstone RM, Adam M, Hammond JR, Orr L, Turbide C. Vesicle formation during reticulocyte maturation. Association of plasma membrane activities with released vesicles (exosomes). The Journal of Biological Chemistry. 1987;**262**:9412-9420

[31] Mathivanan S, Ji H, Simpson RJ. Exosomes: Extracellular organelles important in intercellular communication. Journal of Proteomics. 2010;**73**:1907-1920. DOI: 10.1016/j.jprot.2010.06.006

[32] De Jong OG, Van Balkom BWM, Schiffelers RM, Bouten CVC, Verhaar MC. Extracellular vesicles: Potential roles in regenerative medicine. Frontiers in Immunology. 2014;**5**:608. DOI: 10.3389/fimmu.2014.00608

[33] Thery C, Amigorena S, Raposo G, Clayton A. Isolation and characterization of exosomes from cell culture supernatants and biological fluids. Current Protocols in Cell Biology. 2006;**Chapter 3**:3.22. DOI: 10.1002/0471143030.cb0322s30

[34] Raposo G, Stoorvogel W. Extracellular vesicles: Exosomes, microvesicles, and friends. The Journal of Cell Biology. 2013;**200**:373-383. DOI: 10.1083/jcb.201211138

[35] Bjørge IM, Kim SY, Mano JF, Kalionis B, Chrzanowski W. Extracellular vesicles, exosomes and shedding vesicles in regenerative medicine—A new paradigm for tissue repair. Biomaterials Science. 2018;**6**:60-78. DOI: 10.1039/C7BM00479F

[36] Hsu C, Morohashi Y, Yoshimura S, Manrique-Hoyos N, Jung S, Lauterbach MA, et al. Regulation of exosome secretion by Rab35 and its GTPase-activating proteins TBC1D10A–C. The Journal of Cell Biology. 2010;**189**:223-232. DOI: 10.1083/jcb.200911018

[37] van Niel G, Porto-Carreiro I, Simoes S, Raposo G. Exosomes: A common pathway for a specialized function. The Journal of Biochemistry. 2006;**140**:13-21. DOI: 10.1093/jb/mvj128

[38] Simons M, Raposo G. Exosomes—Vesicular carriers for intercellular communication. Current Opinion in Cell Biology. 2009;**21**:575-581. DOI: 10.1016/j.ceb.2009.03.007

[39] Zitvogel L, Regnault A, Lozier A, Wolfers J, Flament C, Tenza D, et al. Eradication of established murine tumors using a novel cell-free vaccine: Dendritic cell-derived exosomes. Nature Medicine. 1998;**4**:594-600

[40] Van Niel G, Raposo G, Candalh C, Boussac M, Hershberg R, Cerf Bensussan N, et al. Intestinal epithelial cells secrete exosome–like vesicles. Gastroenterology. 2001;**121**:337-349. DOI: 10.1053/gast.2001.26263

[41] Zhang H, Xie Y, Li W, Chibbar R, Xiong S, Xiang J. CD4(+) T cell-released exosomes inhibit CD8(+) cytotoxic T-lymphocyte responses and antitumor immunity. Cellular & Molecular Immunology. 2011;**8**:23-30. DOI: 10.1038/cmi.2010.59

[42] Goldie BJ, Dun MD, Lin M, Smith ND, Verrills NM, Dayas CV, et al. Activity-associated miRNA are packaged in Map1b-enriched exosomes released from depolarized neurons. Nucleic Acids Research. 2014;**42**:9195-9208. DOI: 10.1093/nar/gku594

[43] Xiao H, Lasser C, Shelke GV, Wang J, Radinger M, Lunavat TR, et al. Mast cell exosomes promote lung adenocarcinoma cell proliferation—role of KIT-stem cell factor signaling. Cell Communication and Signaling: CCS. 2014;**12**:64. DOI: 10.1186/s12964-014-0064-8

[44] Pisitkun T, Shen RF, Knepper MA. Identification and proteomic

profiling of exosomes in human urine. Proceedings of the National Academy of Sciences of the United States of America. 2004;**101**:13368-13373. DOI: 10.1073/pnas.0403453101

[45] Keller S, Ridinger J, Rupp AK, Janssen JW, Altevogt P. Body fluid derived exosomes as a novel template for clinical diagnostics. Journal of Translational Medicine. 2011;**9**:86. DOI: 10.1186/1479-5876-9-86

[46] Muller L, Hong C, Stolz DB, Watkins SC, Whiteside TL. Isolation of biologically-active exosomes from human plasma. Journal of Immunological Methods. 2014;**411**:55-65. DOI: 10.1016/j.jim.2014.06.007

[47] Lin J, Li J, Huang B, Liu J, Chen X, Chen X, et al. Exosomes: Novel biomarkers for clinical diagnosis. The Scientific World Journal. 2015;**2015**:1-8. DOI: 10.1155/2015/657086

[48] Valadi H, Ekström K, Bossios A, Sjöstrand M, Lee JJ, Lötvall JO. Exosome-mediated transfer of mRNAs and microRNAs is a novel mechanism of genetic exchange between cells. Nature Cell Biology. 2007;**9**:654-659. DOI: 10.1038/ncb1596

[49] Morhayim J, van de Peppel J, Dudakovic A, Chiba H, van Wijnen AJ, van Leeuwen JP. Molecular characterization of human osteoblast-derived extracellular vesicle mRNA using next-generation sequencing. Biochimica et Biophysica Acta. 2017;**1864**:1133-1141. DOI: 10.1016/j.bbamcr.2017.03.011

[50] Quan L, Wang Y, Liang J, Qiu T, Wang H, Zhang Y, et al. Screening for genes, transcription factors and miRNAs associated with the myogenic and osteogenic differentiation of human adipose tissue-derived stem cells. International Journal of Molecular Medicine. 2016;**38**:1839-1849. DOI: 10.3892/ijmm.2016.2788

[51] Cantaluppi V, Gatti S, Medica D, Figliolini F, Bruno S, Deregibus MC, et al. Microvesicles derived from endothelial progenitor cells protect the kidney from ischemia–reperfusion injury by microRNA-dependent reprogramming of resident renal cells. Kidney International. 2012;**82**:412-427. DOI: 10.1038/ki.2012.105

[52] Aghajani Nargesi A, Lerman LO, Eirin A. Mesenchymal stem cell-derived extracellular vesicles for kidney repair: Current status and looming challenges. Stem Cell Research & Therapy. 2017;**8**(1):273. DOI: 10.1186/s13287-017-0727-7

[53] Ni J, Sun Y, Liu Z. The potential of stem cells and stem cell-derived exosomes in treating cardiovascular diseases. Journal of Cardiovascular Translational Research. 2018;**3**(1):1-11. DOI: 10.1007/s12265-018-9799-8

[54] Tsilioni I, Panagiotidou S, Theoharides TC. Exosomes in neurologic and psychiatric disorders. Clinical Therapeutics. 2014;**36**:882-888. DOI: 10.1016/j.clinthera.2014.05.005

[55] Yamaguchi T, Izumi Y, Nakamura Y, Yamazaki T, Shiota M, Sano S, et al. Repeated remote ischemic conditioning attenuates left ventricular remodeling via exosome-mediated intercellular communication on chronic heart failure after myocardial infarction. International Journal of Cardiology. 2015;**178**:239-246. DOI: 10.1016/j.ijcard.2014.10.144

[56] Lee C, Mitsialis SA, Aslam M, Vitali SH, Vergadi E, Konstantinou G, et al. Exosomes mediate the cytoprotective action of mesenchymal stromal cells on hypoxia-induced pulmonary hypertension. Circulation. 2012;**126**:2601-2611. DOI: 10.1161/CIRCULATIONAHA.112.114173

[57] Burger D, Viñas JL, Akbari S, Dehak H, Knoll W, Gutsol A, et al. Human endothelial colony-forming

cells protect against acute kidney injury. The American Journal of Pathology. 2015;**185**:2309-2323. DOI: 10.1016/j.ajpath.2015.04.010

[58] Hao ZC, Lu J, Wang SZ, Wu H, Zhang YT, Xu SG. Stem cell-derived exosomes: A promising strategy for fracture healing. Cell Proliferation. 2017;**50**(5):1-10. DOI: 10.1111/cpr.12359

[59] Qin Y, Wang L, Gao Z, Chen G, Zhang C. Bone marrow stromal/stem cell-derived extracellular vesicles regulate osteoblast activity and differentiation in vitro and promote bone regeneration in vivo. Scientific Reports. 2016;**50**(5):1-10. DOI: 10.1038/srep21961

[60] Barba M, Cicione C, Bernardini C, Michetti F, Lattanzi W. Adipose-derived mesenchymal cells for bone regereneration: State of the art. BioMed Research International. 2013;**6**:21961. DOI: 10.1155/2013/416391

[61] Zigdon-Giladi H, Michaeli-Geller G, Bick T, Lewinson D, Machtei EE. Human blood-derived endothelial progenitor cells augment vasculogenesis and osteogenesis. Journal of Clinical Periodontology. 2015;**42**:89-95. DOI: 10.1111/jcpe.12325

[62] Goerke SM, Obermeyer J, Plaha J, Stark GB, Finkenzeller G. Endothelial progenitor cells from peripheral blood support bone regeneration by provoking an angiogenic response. Microvascular Research. 2015;**98**:40-47. DOI: 10.1016/j.mvr.2014.12.001

[63] Yin P, Lv H, Li Y, Deng Y, Zhang L, Tang P. Exosome-mediated genetic information transfer, a missing piece of osteoblast–osteoclast communication puzzle. Frontiers in Endocrinology. 2017;**8**:336. DOI: 10.3389/fendo.2017.00336

[64] Inose H, Ochi H, Kimura A, Fujita K, Xu R, Sato S, et al. A microRNA regulatory mechanism of osteoblast differentiation. Proceedings of repair in a mouse model. Arthritis and Rheumatism. 2009;**60**:813-823. DOI: 10.1002/art.24330

[65] Martins M, Ribeiro D, Martins A, Reis RL, Neves NM. Extracellular vesicles derived from osteogenically induced human bone marrow mesenchymal stem cells can modulate lineage commitment. Stem Cell Reports. 2016;**6**:284-291. DOI: 10.1016/j.stemcr.2016.01.001

[66] Pegtel DM, Cosmopoulos K, Thorley-Lawson DA, van Eijndhoven MAJ, Hopmans ES, Lindenberg JL, et al. Functional delivery of viral miRNAs via exosomes. Proceedings of the National Academy of Sciences. 2010;**107**:6328-6333. DOI: 10.1073/pnas.0914843107

[67] Xu JF, Yang GH, Pan XH, Zhang SJ, Zhao C, Qiu BS, et al. Altered microRNA expression profile in exosomes during osteogenic differentiation of human bone marrow-derived mesenchymal stem cells. PLoS One. 2014;**9**:e114627. DOI: 10.1371/journal.pone.0114627

[68] Wei J, Li H, Wang S, Li T, Fan J, Liang X, et al. Let-7 enhances osteogenesis and bone formation while repressing adipogenesis of human stromal/mesenchymal stem cells by regulating HMGA2. Stem Cells and Development. 2014;**23**:1452-1463. DOI: 10.1089/scd.2013.0600

[69] Furuta T, Miyaki S, Ishitobi H, Ogura T, Kato Y, Kamei N, et al. Mesenchymal stem cell-derived exosomes promote fracture healing in a mouse model. Stem Cells Translational Medicine. 2016;**5**:1620-1630. DOI: 10.5966/sctm.2015-0285

[70] Kitaori T, Ito H, Schwarz EM, Tsutsumi R, Yoshitomi H, Oishi S, et al. Stromal cell-derived factor 1/CXCR4 signaling is critical for the

recruitment of mesenchymal stem cells to the fracture site during skeletal repair in a mouse model. Arthritis and Rheumatism. 2009;**60**:813-823. DOI: 10.1002/art.24330

[71] Ishikawa M, Ito H, Kitaori T, Murata K, Shibuya H, Furu M, et al. MCP/CCR2 signaling is essential for recruitment of mesenchymal progenitor cells during the early phase of fracture healing. PLoS One. 2014;**9**:e104954. DOI: 10.1371/journal.pone.0104954

[72] Wang X, Omar O, Vazirisani F, Thomsen P, Ekström K. Mesenchymal stem cell-derived exosomes have altered microRNA profiles and induce osteogenic differentiation depending on the stage of differentiation. PLoS One. 2018;**13**:e193059. DOI: 10.1371/journal.pone.0193059

[73] Bakhshandeh B, Hafizi M, Ghaemi N, Soleimani M. Down-regulation of miRNA-221 triggers osteogenic differentiation in human stem cells. Biotechnology Letters. 2012;**34**:1579-1587. DOI: 10.1007/s10529-012-0934-3

[74] Baglìo SR, Devescovi V, Granchi D, Baldini N. MicroRNA expression profiling of human bone marrow mesenchymal stem cells during osteogenic differentiation reveals Osterix regulation by miR-31. Gene. 2013;**527**:321-331. DOI: 10.1016/j.gene.2013.06.021

[75] Sun Y, Xu L, Huang S, Hou Y, Liu Y, Chan K, et al. Mir-21 overexpressing mesenchymal stem cells accelerate fracture healing in a rat closed femur fracture model. BioMed Research International. 2015;**2015**:1-9. DOI: 10.1155/2015/412327

[76] Huang C, Geng J, Wei X, Zhang R, Jiang S. MiR-144-3p regulates osteogenic differentiation and proliferation of murine mesenchymal stem cells by specifically targetingSmad4. FEBS Letters. 2016;**590**:795-807. DOI: 10.1002/1873-3468.12112

[77] Cong R, Tao K, Fu P, Lou L, Zhu Y, Chen S, et al. MicroRNA218 promotes prostaglandin E2 to inhibit osteogenic differentiation in synovial mesenchymal stem cells by targeting 15hydroxyprostaglandin dehydrogenase [NAD(+)]. Molecular Medicine Reports. 2017;**16**:9347-9354. DOI: 10.3892/mmr.2017.7795

[78] Chen C, Cheng P, Xie H, Zhou H, Wu X, Liao E, et al. MiR-503 regulates osteoclastogenesis via targeting RANK. Journal of Bone and Mineral Research. 2014;**29**:338-347. DOI: 10.1002/jbmr.2032

[79] Xie Y, Chen Y, Zhang L, Ge W, Tang P. The roles of bone-derived exosomes and exosomal microRNAs in regulating bone remodelling. Journal of Cellular and Molecular Medicine. 2017;**21**:1033-1041. DOI: 10.1111/jcmm.13039

[80] Xu Q, Cui Y, Luan J, Zhou X, Li H, Han J. Exosomes from C2C12 myoblasts enhance osteogenic differentiation of MC3T3-E1 pre-osteoblasts by delivering miR-27a-3p. Biochemical and Biophysical Research Communications. 2018;**498**:32-37. DOI: 10.1016/j.bbrc.2018.02.144

[81] Li D, Liu J, Guo B, Liang C, Dang L, Lu C, et al. Osteoclast-derived exosomal miR-214-3p inhibits osteoblastic bone formation. Nature Communications. 2016;**7**:10872. DOI: 10.1038/ncomms10872

[82] Li W, Liu Y, Zhang P, Tang Y, Zhou M, Jiang W, et al. Tissue-engineered bone immobilized with human adipose stem cells-derived exosomes promotes bone regeneration. ACS Applied Materials & Interfaces. 2018;**10**:5240-5254. DOI: 10.1021/acsami.7b17620

[83] Wang K, Xu L, Rui Y, Huang S, Lin S, Xiong J, et al. The effects of secretion

factors from umbilical cord derived mesenchymal stem cells on osteogenic differentiation of mesenchymal stem cells. PLoS One. 2015;**10**:e120593. DOI: 10.1371/journal.pone.0120593

[84] Qi X, Zhang J, Yuan H, Xu Z, Li Q, Niu X, et al. Exosomes secreted by human-induced pluripotent stem cell-derived mesenchymal stem cells repair critical-sized bone defects through enhanced angiogenesis and osteogenesis in osteoporotic rats. International Journal of Biological Sciences. 2016;**12**:836-849. DOI: 10.7150/ijbs.14809

[85] Zhang Y, Xie RL, Croce CM, Stein JL, Lian JB, van Wijnen AJ, et al. A program of microRNAs controls osteogenic lineage progression by targeting transcription factor Runx2. Proceedings of the National Academy of Sciences. 2011;**108**:9863-9868. DOI: 10.1073/pnas.1018493108

[86] Zhang Y, Xie R, Gordon J, LeBlanc K, Stein JL, Lian JB, et al. Control of mesenchymal lineage progression by MicroRNAs targeting skeletal gene regulators Trps1 and Runx2. Journal of Biological Chemistry. 2012;**287**:21926-21935. DOI: 10.1074/jbc.M112.340398

[87] Deng Y, Zhou H, Gu P, Fan X. Repair of canine medial orbital bone defects with miR-31-modified bone marrow mesenchymal stem cells. Investigative Ophthalmology & Visual Science. 2014;**55**:6016-6023. DOI: 10.1167/iovs.14-14977

[88] Ghosh-Choudhury N. Requirement of BMP-2-induced phosphatidylinositol 3-kinase and Akt serine/threonine kinase in osteoblast differentiation and Smad-dependent BMP-2 gene transcription. Journal of Biological Chemistry. 2002;**277**:33361-33368. DOI: 10.1074/jbc.M205053200

[89] Suzuki E, Ochiai-Shino H, Aoki H, Onodera S, Saito A, Saito A, et al. Akt activation is required for TGF-β1-induced osteoblast differentiation of MC3T3-E1 pre-osteoblasts. PLoS One. 2014;**9**:e112566. DOI: 10.1371/journal.pone.0112566

[90] Shabbir A, Cox A, Rodriguez-Menocal L, Salgado M, Badiavas EV. Mesenchymal stem cell exosomes induce proliferation and migration of normal and chronic wound fibroblasts, and enhance angiogenesis in vitro. Stem Cells and Development. 2015;**24**:1635-1647. DOI: 10.1089/scd.2014.0316

[91] Zhang J, Liu X, Li H, Chen C, Hu B, Niu X, et al. Exosomes/tricalcium phosphate combination scaffolds can enhance bone regeneration by activating the PI3K/Akt signaling pathway. Stem Cell Research & Therapy. 2016;**7**. DOI: 10.1186/s13287-016-0391-3

[92] Trohatou O, Zagoura D, Bitsika V, Pappa KI, Antsaklis A, Anagnou NP, et al. Sox2 suppression by miR-21 governs human mesenchymal stem cell properties. Stem Cells Translational Medicine. 2014;**3**:54-68. DOI: 10.5966/sctm.2013-0081

[93] Meng YB, Li X, Li ZY, Zhao J, Yuan XB, Ren Y, et al. microRNA-21 promotes osteogenic differentiation of mesenchymal stem cells by the PI3K/beta-catenin pathway. Journal of Orthopaedic Research. 2015;**33**:957-964. DOI: 10.1002/jor.22884

[94] Liu X, Li Q, Niu X, Hu B, Chen S, Song W, et al. Exosomes secreted from human-induced pluripotent stem cell-derived mesenchymal stem cells prevent osteonecrosis of the femoral head by promoting angiogenesis. International Journal of Biological Sciences. 2017;**13**:232-244. DOI: 10.7150/ijbs.16951

[95] Leucht P, Lee S, Yim N. Wnt signaling and bone regeneration: Can't have one without the other.

Biomaterials. 2018;**3**(15):S0142-9612(18)30196-0. DOI: 10.1016/j.biomaterials.2018.03.029

[96] Lu Z, Chen Y, Dunstan C, Roohani-Esfahani S, Zreiqat H. Priming adipose stem cells with tumor necrosis factor-alpha preconditioning potentiates their exosome efficacy for bone regeneration. Tissue Engineering Part A. 2017;**23**:1212-1220. DOI: 10.1089/ten.tea.2016.0548

[97] Zhang B, Wu X, Zhang X, Sun Y, Yan Y, Shi H, et al. Human umbilical cord mesenchymal stem cell exosomes enhance angiogenesis through the Wnt4/beta-catenin pathway. Stem Cells Translational Medicine. 2015;**4**:513-522. DOI: 10.5966/sctm.2014-0267

[98] McBride JD, Rodriguez-Menocal L, Guzman W, Candanedo A, Garcia-Contreras M, Badiavas EV. Bone marrow mesenchymal stem cell-derived CD63(+) exosomes transport Wnt3a exteriorly and enhance dermal fibroblast proliferation, migration, and angiogenesis In vitro. Stem Cells and Development. 2017;**26**:1384-1398. DOI: 10.1089/scd.2017.0087

[99] Huynh N, VonMoss L, Smith D, Rahman I, Felemban MF, Zuo J, et al. Characterization of regulatory extracellular vesicles from osteoclasts. Journal of Dental Research. 2016;**95**:673-679. DOI: 10.1177/0022034516633189

[100] Deng L, Wang Y, Peng Y, Wu Y, Ding Y, Jiang Y, et al. Osteoblast-derived microvesicles: A novel mechanism for communication between osteoblasts and osteoclasts. Bone. 2015;**79**:37-42. DOI: 10.1016/j.bone.2015.05.022

[101] Chen X, Zhi X, Yin Z, Li X, Qin L, Qiu Z, et al. 18β-Glycyrrhetinic acid inhibits osteoclastogenesis in vivo and in vitro by blocking RANKL-mediated RANK–TRAF6 interactions and NF-κB and MAPK signaling pathways. Frontiers in Pharmacology. 2018;**9**:647. DOI: 10.3389/fphar.2018.00647

[102] Narayanan R, Huang C, Ravindran S. Hijacking the cellular mail: Exosome mediated differentiation of mesenchymal stem cells. Stem Cells International. 2016;**2016**:1-11. DOI: 10.1155/2016/3808674

[103] Zhao L, Jiang S, Hantash BM. Transforming growth factor beta1 induces osteogenic differentiation of murine bone marrow stromal cells. Tissue Engineering. Part A. 2010;**16**:725-733. DOI: 10.1089/ten.TEA.2009.0495

[104] Lamplot JD, Qin J, Nan G, Wang J, Liu X, Yin L, et al. BMP9 signaling in stem cell differentiation and osteogenesis. American Journal of Stem Cells. 2013;**2**:1-21

[105] Minardi S, Pandolfi L, Taraballi F, Wang X, De Rosa E, Mills ZD, et al. Enhancing vascularization through the controlled release of platelet-derived growth factor-BB. ACS Applied Materials & Interfaces. 2017;**9**:14566-14575. DOI: 10.1021/acsami.6b13760

[106] Al Rifai O, Chow J, Lacombe J, Julien C, Faubert D, Susan-Resiga D, et al. Proprotein convertase furin regulates osteocalcin and bone endocrine function. Journal of Clinical Investigation. 2017;**127**:4104-4117. DOI: 10.1172/JCI93437

[107] Feng JQ, Ward LM, Liu S, Lu Y, Xie Y, Yuan B, et al. Loss of DMP1 causes rickets and osteomalacia and identifies a role for osteocytes in mineral metabolism. Nature Genetics. 2006;**38**:1310-1315. DOI: 10.1038/ng1905

[108] Ramachandran A, Ravindran S, Huang C, George A. TGF beta receptor II interacting protein-1, an intracellular protein has an extracellular role as a modulator of matrix mineralization. Scientific Reports. 2016;**6**. DOI: 10.1038/srep37885

[109] Pethő A, Chen Y, George A. Exosomes in extracellular matrix bone biology. Current Osteoporosis Reports. 2018;**16**:58-64. DOI: 10.1007/s11914-018-0419-y

[110] Li C, Sunderic K, Nicoll SB, Wang S. Downregulation of heat shock protein 70 impairs osteogenic and chondrogenic differentiation in human mesenchymal stem cells. Scientific Reports. 2018;**8**(1):553. DOI: 10.1038/s41598-017-18541-1

[111] Flanagan M, Li C, Dietrich MA, Richard M, Yao S. Downregulation of heat shock protein B8 decreases osteogenic differentiation potential of dental pulp stem cells during in vitro proliferation. Cell Proliferation. 2018;**51**:e12420. DOI: 10.1111/cpr.12420

[112] Lankford KL, Arroyo EJ, Nazimek K, Bryniarski K, Askenase PW, Kocsis JD. Intravenously delivered mesenchymal stem cell-derived exosomes target M2-type macrophages in the injured spinal cord. PLoS One. 2018;**13**:e190358. DOI: 10.1371/journal.pone.0190358

[113] Zhang B, Yeo RWY, Lai RC, Sim EWK, Chin KC, Lim SK. Mesenchymal stromal cell exosome–enhanced regulatory T-cell production through an antigen-presenting cell–mediated pathway. Cytotherapy. 2018;**20**(5):687-696. DOI: 10.1016/j.jcyt.2018.02.372

[114] Nassar W, El-Ansary M, Sabry D, Mostafa MA, Fayad T, Kotb E, et al. Umbilical cord mesenchymal stem cells derived extracellular vesicles can safely ameliorate the progression of chronic kidney diseases. Biomaterials Research. 2016;**20**:21. DOI: 10.1186/s40824-016-0068-0

[115] Gardiner C, Vizio DD, Sahoo S, Théry C, Witwer KW, Wauben M, et al. Techniques used for the isolation and characterization of extracellular vesicles: Results of a worldwide survey. Journal of Extracellular Vesicles. 2016;**5**:32945. DOI: 10.3402/jev.v5.32945

[116] Ahrlund-Richter L, De Luca M, Marshak DR, Munsie M, Veiga A, Rao M. Isolation and production of cells suitable for human therapy: Challenges ahead. Cell Stem Cell. 2009;**4**:20-26. DOI: 10.1016/j.stem.2008.11.012

[117] Chen AK, Chen X, Choo ABH, Reuveny S, Oh SKW. Critical microcarrier properties affecting the expansion of undifferentiated human embryonic stem cells. Stem Cell Research. 2011;**7**:97-111. DOI: 10.1016/j.scr.2011.04.007

[118] Li P, Kaslan M, Lee SH, Yao J, Gao Z. Progress in exosome isolation techniques. Theranostics. 2017;**7**:789-804. DOI: 10.7150/thno.18133

[119] Beaudeux JL, Peynet J, Flourie F, Keddad K, Delattre J, Rousselet F, et al. Discrepancies between lipoprotein(a) concentrations in icteric sera measured by immunonephelometry and electroimmunodiffusion. Clinical Biochemistry. 1994;**27**:7-11

[120] Wen Y, Chang Y, Lin L, Liao P. Collection of in vivo-like liver cell secretome with alternative sample enrichment method using a hollow fiber bioreactor culture system combined with tangential flow filtration for secretomics analysis. Analytica Chimica Acta. 2011;**684**:81-88. DOI: 10.1016/j.aca.2010.10.040

[121] Suárez H, Gámez-Valero A, Reyes R, López-Martín S, Rodríguez MJ, Carrascosa JL, et al. A bead-assisted flow cytometry method for the semi-quantitative analysis of extracellular vesicles. Scientific Reports. 2017;**7**(1):11271. DOI: 10.1038/s41598-017-11249-2

[122] Du T, Ju G, Wu S, Cheng Z, Cheng J, Zou X, et al. Microvesicles derived from human Wharton's jelly mesenchymal

stem cells promote human renal cancer cell growth and aggressiveness through induction of hepatocyte growth factor. PLoS One. 2014;**9**:e96836. DOI: 10.1371/journal.pone.0096836

[123] Peak TC, Praharaj PP, Panigrahi GK, Doyle M, Su Y, Schlaepfer IR, et al. Exosomes secreted by placental stem cells selectively inhibit growth of aggressive prostate cancer cells. Biochemical and Biophysical Research Communications. 2018;**499**(4):1004-1010. DOI: 10.1016/j.bbrc.2018.04.038

[124] Qi J, Zhou Y, Jiao Z, Wang X, Zhao Y, Li Y, et al. Exosomes derived from human bone marrow mesenchymal stem cells promote tumor growth through hedgehog signaling pathway. Cellular Physiology and Biochemistry. 2017;**42**:2242-2254. DOI: 10.1159/000479998

[125] Wang J, Hendrix A, Hernot S, Lemaire M, De Bruyne E, Van Valckenborgh E, et al. Bone marrow stromal cell-derived exosomes as communicators in drug resistance in multiple myeloma cells. Blood. 2014;**124**:555-566. DOI: 10.1182/blood-2014-03-562439

[126] Roccaro AM, Sacco A, Maiso P, Azab AK, Tai Y, Reagan M, et al. BM mesenchymal stromal cell–derived exosomes facilitate multiple myeloma progression. Journal of Clinical Investigation. 2013;**123**:1542-1555. DOI: 10.1172/JCI66517

[127] Umezu T, Imanishi S, Azuma K, Kobayashi C, Yoshizawa S, Ohyashiki K, et al. Replenishing exosomes from older bone marrow stromal cells with miR-340 inhibits myeloma-related angiogenesis. Blood Advances. 2017;**1**:812-823. DOI: 10.1182/bloodadvances.2016003251

Chapter 4

Role of Inflammatory Factors in Regulation of Osteogenesis in Tissue-Engineered Bone

Yandong Mu, Lu Yang, Chenglong Li and Wei Qing

Abstract

It was traditionally considered that the inhibition of inflammatory reaction is necessary for osteogenesis, but the latest issue argued inflammation is unavoidable in the process of bone trauma, and physiological inflammatory reaction is essential to achieve bone formation. Tissue-engineered bone graft is not only associated with osteoblast-related cells; the inflammatory reaction is the initial physiological process, mainly with neutrophil infiltration, which secretes MCP-1, IL-8, and other chemokines and further promotes dendritic cells, lymphocytes, and mononuclear macrophages to move in. The activation pathways of macrophages have a direct effect on the outcome of the inflammatory reaction and the healing, which are divided into the classical approach (M1) and the alternative approach (M2). The M1 pathway secretes IL-1 beta, IL-6, TNF-α, and other pro-inflammatory factors, while the M2 pathway secretes arginase, IL-1Ra, IL-4, and other anti-inflammatory cytokines, also with bone-healing-related growth factors, which promote homing of bone mesenchymal stem cells (bMSCs).

Keywords: tissue-engineered bone, osteogenesis, inflammatory factors, immune cells, osteoimmunology

1. Introduction

The human bone tissue has a certain self-healing ability, but for large bone defects, which measures up to more than 6–8 mm cannot self-repair. Currently, the main method for the treatment of large bone defects includes autograft and allograft, distraction osteogenesis, synthetic or natural material implanting, and bone tissue engineering [1–3]. Each method has its own advantages and disadvantages. At present, the most commonly used autograft or allogeneic bone graft has good osteogenesis, but autologous bone transplantation can cause greater trauma to the donor site, while allograft bone will inevitably have an immune response or a potential biological safety risk [4–7]. Although distraction osteogenesis can avoid the trauma of the donor area, the course of treatment is too long [8]. Synthetic or natural materials are widely distributed, but their biocompatibility is low and cannot participate in normal physiological metabolism [9, 10].

Bone tissue engineering is a new combination of life science and material science to establish human bone tissue reconstruction and recovery; its basic elements include seed cells, scaffold materials, growth factors, and biomechanics microenvironment. When amplification of stem cells cultured in vitro adsorbed on the biocompatibility biological material that can be absorbed by the body transplanted to the damaged bone site, accompanied by biological scaffold being absorbed, osteogenic differentiation, and secretion of matrix and mineralization occur, the formation of new bone and reconstruction take place [11]. The advantages of bone tissue engineering include no extra supply area damage, no graft rejection, and no risk of the spread of the disease [12], but currently this technique can only be able to regenerate and repair some tiny bone defects, and large bone defects still remain to be solved, while the main challenge is without an independent blood supply system, which provides nutrients and growth factor; also metabolite is transported by very limited diffusion and osmosis [13, 14].

Seed cells need to meet a wide range of sources, non-immunogenicity, and a strong ability to differentiate [15]. Currently, research is mainly focused on embryonic stem cells, bone marrow mesenchymal stem cells, dental pulp stem cells, and induced pluripotent stem cells [16]. Biological scaffold materials provide space for cell adhesion, proliferation, and differentiation and promote tissue regeneration. According to their source, biological scaffolds can be divided into natural material scaffolds and synthetic material scaffolds. Natural material scaffolds include natural polymer materials, natural bone-derived materials, and natural coral bone-derived materials which advantages include widely distributed, good degradation performance, and good biocompatibility; however, disadvantages cover low mechanical strength, high brittleness, and no bone induction. Research shows that cells can receive enough nutrients and oxygen by diffusion with the distance from the capillary by 20–200 μm but cannot meet the metabolic needs beyond this distance. With the increase of scaffold material size, the internal cell microenvironment, nutrition, and oxygen gradient decreased [17, 18]. Besides, isothermal conditions, proper pH value, and adequate nutrition supply are also important factors restricting the repair of large bone defects by tissue-engineered bone.

Growth factors regulate cell division, matrix synthesis, and tissue differentiation by autocrine and paracrine [19]. Study confirmed that growth factor is related to osteogenesis induced by bone morphogenetic protein, transforming growth factor beta, platelet-derived growth factor, and insulin-like growth factor, while bone morphogenetic protein in bone tissue engineering has the most significant effect [20]; an experiment proved that its application combined with vascular endothelial growth factor shows extraordinary effect of bone healing [21].

Once the tissue engineering materials are implanted in the area, the allogenic reaction is quickly triggered, showing aseptic inflammation, and starts the tissue repair function. Tissue-engineered bone graft is not only associated with osteoblast-related cells; the inflammatory reaction is the first physiological process [22, 23]. Tissue engineering bone implantation is accompanied by an early inflammatory reaction, mainly with macrophages and neutrophil infiltration, which secretes MCP-1, IL-8, and other chemokines and further promotes dendritic cells, lymphocytes, and mononuclear macrophages to move in [24, 25]. As time goes on, neutrophils are gradually apoptotic and phagocytic by macrophages. The activation of macrophages has a direct effect on the outcome of the inflammatory reaction and the healing [26]. The activation pathway is divided into the classical approach (M1) and the alternative approach (M2). The M1 pathway secretes IL-1 beta, IL-6, TNF-α, a pro-inflammatory factor, while the M2 pathway secretes arginase, IL-1Ra, IL-4, and other anti-inflammatory cytokines, also with bone-healing-related growth factors that promote homing of bMSCs [27].

Pathological inflammatory reaction can lead to failure of fibrous wrapping and bony binding. Chemokines and cytokines produced by physiological inflammatory reaction, such as MCP-1 and VEGF, can promote osteogenesis and angiogenesis of bMSCs. Traditionally, the inhibition of inflammatory reaction is an important means of osteogenesis, but now, it has a deeper understanding of inflammatory response. Avoiding inflammatory reaction cannot achieve its goal; physiological inflammatory reaction is essential to achieve bone formation [28, 29].

Inflammation is unavoidable in the process of bone trauma; it is considered that inflammatory reaction plays a crucial role in the process of bone healing. The concept of osteoimmunology is attracting more and more attention. The immune system plays an important role in the skeletal system, and studies have shown that many diseases are closely related to the bone immune system. Kayal, R A suggests that periodontitis is closely related to bone immunity; in the fight against foreign microbes, inflammatory cells and inflammatory mediators also activate the protease to induce matrix degradation, resulting in bone resorption [30]. Kamiya, N found the active phase of Perthes disease (LCPD), and the increased IL-6 in the synovial fluid of the synovial joint was detected [31]. Cafiero, C found that chronic kidney disease is accompanied by abnormal verification and skeletal abnormalities, which may be related to the increased expression of nuclear factor kappa B receptor-activating factor ligand (RANKL) [32]. Metzger et al. [33] have found that inflammatory bowel disease (IBD) causes the inflammatory state of the body to cause bone loss. Spinal arthropathy and progressive ossification are also diseases caused by an abnormal bone immune system. HIV-infected persons show different degrees of bone-healing disorders. This also explains to some extent that the defects of the immune system have an important impact on bone healing [34]. What are the important inflammatory factors involved in the process and the mechanism involved in osteogenesis? This article provides a framework.

2. Host initial immune response

Tissue-engineered bone graft always accompanies with implant surgery; at the same time, tissue damage is followed by a series of biochemical reactions at nanosecond level on the surface of biomaterial, which includes activation of coagulation, complement system, and immune system. Every step of these reactions significantly determines the later physiological processes; we believe that early regulation, especially initial immune regulation, is potent for tissue prognosis.

2.1 Transient protein adsorption of biomaterial implanting

When implant surgery carried on, blood coagulation factors such as fibrinogen and factor XII can be absorbed on the biomaterial surface spontaneously, which initiate coagulation cascade; also with activation of platelets, tissue factor generated by damaged tissue amplifies this process. Complement is also capable of absorbing biomaterial, especially C3 and C3b. The complement synergistically interacts with coagulation cascade, which takes advantage of adherence of platelets. Immunoregulatory function has also been found in complement, which triggers leukocyte activation and mast cell degranulation [35, 36].

Other attachment proteins include fibronectin and vitronectin in the extracellular matrix, which have the ability to activate inflammatory response and also promote osteoblast adherence. It is also worth mentioning that danger signals, which named alarmins consist of ATP, uric acid, heat shock proteins, and so on, may activate immune cells through pattern recognition receptors (PRRs), mainly with Toll-like receptors [37].

2.2 Acute inflammatory cell infiltration and pro-inflammatory factor release

Once the tissue damage occurs, polymorphonuclear leukocytes (PMNs) migrate to the damage site and initiate acute inflammation reflection. PMNs' activation is associated with integrin and PRR attached on the surface protein of biomaterial [38]. PMNs secrete a series of cytokines, which usually lead to acute inflammation; IL-6, IL-8, and CCL2 are important factors which lead to proteolytic enzymes and ROS autocrine. IL-6 is produced by osteoblasts and stimulates osteoclasts to promote bone resorption. It acts by binding to soluble IL-6 receptor (sIL-6R) present in serum and acts as an agonist to promote ubiquitin/IL-6 signal transduction. IL-6 in the body has a role in regulating immune activity, acute phase reactions, and hematopoietic activity (**Figure 1**). CCL2, also named as monocyte chemotactic protein 1 (MCP-1), has a strong chemotaxis function of recruiting monocytes which transfer into macrophages when reaching the inflammation site, also along with dendritic cells and lymphocytes. With continuous activation, PMNs undergo apoptosis within 2 days and are swallowed by macrophages. As the most diverse histiocytes, macrophages play an important role in the process of tissue remodeling [39]. It shows remarkable functional plasticity and plays a very different role in physiological and pathological environment. At present, macrophages are divided into classically activated (M1) and alternatively activated (M2) phenotypes, which are similar to Th1/Th2 subsets of helper T cells. Interferon γ (IFN-γ), lipopolysaccharide (LPS), and tumor necrosis factor-α (TNF-α) can activate the M1 phenotype, which subsequently secretes large quantities of pro-inflammatory cytokines such as IL-1β, IL-6, IL-23, TNF-α, arginine, inducible nitric oxide synthase (iNOS), and reactive oxygen species (ROS). In addition, lymphocytes, especially T cells, are proved to have an enhancement effect on macrophages [40–42].

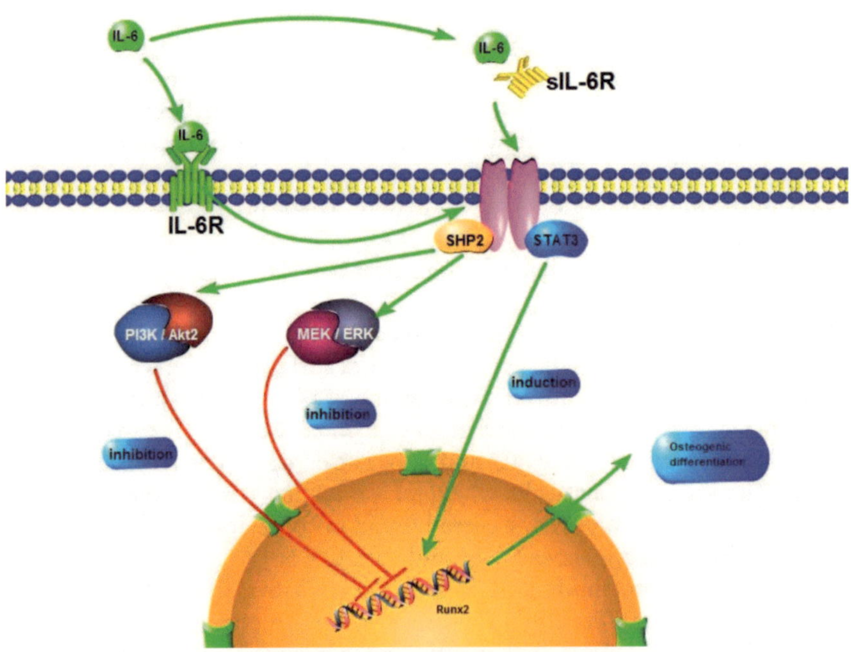

Figure 1.
IL-6 can bind to soluble IL-6 receptor (sIL-6R) present in serum and exerts its effect. IL-6 can activate two major signaling pathways, SHP2/MEK/ERK and SHP2/PI3K/Akt2, as well as JAK/STAT3 signaling pathways. IL-6 negatively regulates osteoblast differentiation through SHP2/MEK2/ERK and SHP2/PI3K/Akt2 pathways and positively regulates osteogenic differentiation through the JAK/STAT3 pathway.

2.3 BMSCs' chemotaxis

Endogenous bone marrow mesenchymal stem cells (BMSCs) have the ability to migrate spontaneously to the injured site and participate in the repair of corresponding tissues, and their directional migration depends on the interaction between chemoattractant molecules expressed locally and the corresponding receptors on the cell surface. After tissue injury, endogenous BMSCs moved out of the bone marrow, entered peripheral blood circulation and migrated to injured tissue, adhered to target vascular endothelial cells, and passed through the extracellular matrix barrier and get to the injured tissue to repair [43–46]. BMSCs are also capable to secrete a variety of growth factors that are conducive to the differentiation of hematopoietic stem cells such as IL-6, IL-11, granulocyte colony-stimulating factor (G-CSF), stem cell factor, and so on. Recent studies suggest that the main factors of chemotactic bone marrow mesenchymal stem cells are as follows: (1) Stromal cell-derived factor 1 (SDF-1) (**Figure 2**) can obviously enhance the chemotaxis function of BMSCs, the number of which is proportional to the gradient of SDF-1 concentration. Study showed that the expression of SDF-1 was significantly increased after injury of the myocardium, liver, kidney, lung, and skin to form a difference in the concentration gradient with the bone marrow, so that it may play an important role in the directional migration of bone marrow mesenchymal stem cells [47]. (2) Monocyte chemoattractant protein 1 (MCP-1)

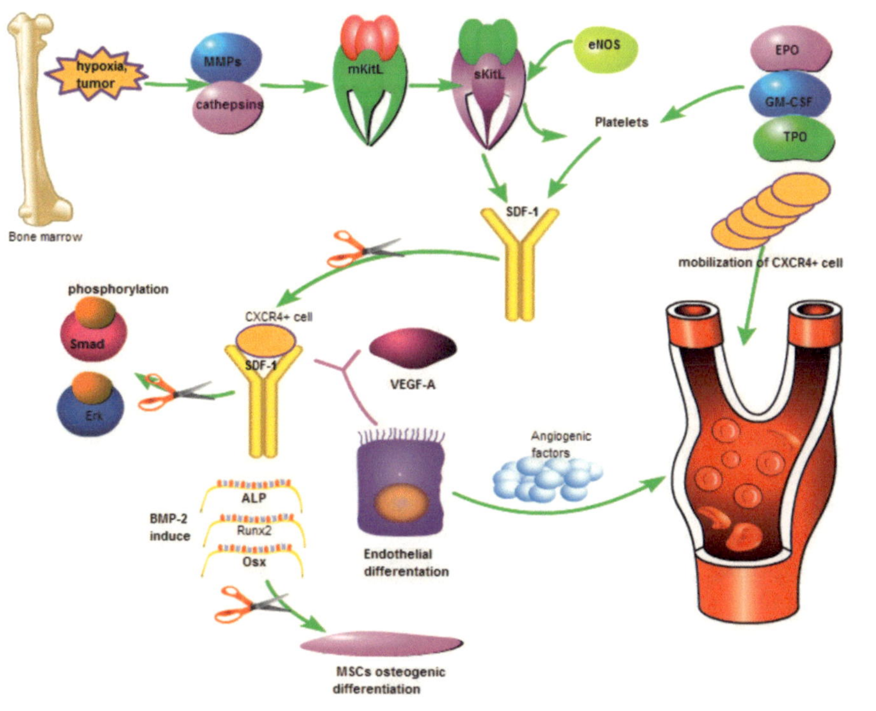

Figure 2.
Regulation of neovascularization by SDF-1. The chemokine SDF-1 is produced by hypoxic conditions, vascular injury, or tumors and is released in the circulation. SDF-1 signaling induces a complex remodeling of the BM microenvironment involving proteases, kit-ligand (KitL), and NO production, leading to mobilization of CXCR4+ angiogenic cells. Ultimately, SDF-1 expression in the neo-angiogenic niche recruits CXCR4+ cells and mediates their proper retention, differentiation, and pro-angiogenic activities in coordination with other angiogenic factors such as VEGF-A. Both PI3K/Akt and MAPK/ERK transduction pathways are involved in the enhancement of MSC migration induced via CXCR4. MSC migration was inhibited by AMD3100, LY294002, PD98059, and p38MAPK inhibitor (SB203580). Perturbing the SDF-1/CXCR4 signal axis affected the BMP2-induced osteogenic differentiation in mouse bone marrow-derived MSCs.

is a multifunctional chemokine that plays an important role in inflammatory response, injury repair, and neovascularization. Recent studies have shown that MCP-1 can promote the migration of bone marrow mesenchymal stem cells to the injured site in animal models of cerebral ischemia injury [48]. (3) Granulocyte colony-stimulating factor (G-CSF): in recent years, it has been found that G-CSF can mobilize BMSCs into blood circulation and migrate to the injury site which can be blocked by antibodies against CXCR4. Whereas BMSCs also express CXCR4, G-CSF is mobilized through a similar mechanism that remains to be further confirmed [49]. (4) Mesenchymal metalloproteinase-9 (MMP-9): Endothelial cells, fibroblasts, and inflammatory cells release interstitial metalloproteinases during inflammation or hypoxia. Recent studies have revealed that BMSCs regulate the recovery, proliferation, and differentiation of hematopoietic stem cells and endothelial stem cells through the release of soluble Kit-ligand (sKitl) mediated by mesenchymal metalloproteinase-9 to promote the migration of BMSCs by mobilizing bone marrow mesenchymal stem cells into the peripheral blood [50, 51].

3. Host anti-inflammatory phase and healing

In the late stage of acute inflammation, the polymorphonuclear granulocytes were swallowed by macrophages, and the tissues were mainly infiltrated by macrophages. Macrophages play a bidirectional role in the process of disease and tissue remodeling according to their different polarization function. Whether this action is positive or harmful depends on the transformation and balance between the polarization state of macrophage and the polarization state of M1/M2. For tissue engineering materials, the polarization of macrophages plays an important role in the function of macrophages. In view of the acute inflammatory response and infiltration of inflammatory macrophages that cannot be avoided in the early stages of implantation of bone implants, therefore, promoting the rapid and effective transformation of peri-implant inflammatory macrophages to M2 macrophages may be more helpful to promote bone healing and long-term stability of implants [42, 52, 53]. Good bone immune microenvironment can effectively promote osteogenic differentiation, while poor bone immune microenvironment can inhibit osteogenic differentiation, resulting in the formation of fibrous envelope.

3.1 Subside of acute inflammation and release of anti-inflammatory factors

Macrophages secrete a large number of bioactive factors under the certain action of tissue microenvironment. The types and secretion of these factors are closely related to the polarization and functional state of macrophages. Although there is still controversy, macrophages are divided into two major phenotypes: classically activated (M1) and alternatively activated (M2). This is very similar to the Th1/Th2 subsets of helper T cells. M1 macrophages are activated by pro-inflammatory signals such as interferon γ (IFN-γ) alone or in conjunction with lipopolysaccharide (LPS) and tumor necrosis factor-α (TNF-α) in which main surface markers were CD80 and CCR7, also known as pro-inflammatory macrophages, which secreted pro-inflammatory cytokines such as TNF-α, IL-1 β, arginine, inducible nitric oxide synthase (iNOS), and reactive oxygen species (ROS), but rarely secreted anti-inflammatory factors such as IL-10. Its main role is to kill bacteria and other pathogens and participate in the Th1-type inflammation as both the initial and effector cells. The main markers of M2 macrophages are CD163 and CD206, also known as repair macrophages. Macrophage differentiation to M2 was induced by alternative pathways such as IL-4, IL-10, and an immune complex (IC). M2 subtype can release IL-10,

IL-4, vascular endothelial growth factor (VEGF), platelet-derived growth factor BB (PDGF-BB), and transforming growth factor beta (TGF-β), which are beneficial to the formation and remodeling of new bone and extra cellular matrix (ECM) remodeling and angiogenesis [54–58]. The concentrations of pro-inflammatory factors such as IL-1 β, IL-6, and TNF-α (**Figure 3**) increased rapidly after trauma in order to initiate inflammation and bone repair in physiological environment and then gradually decreased and disappeared within 72 hours.

3.2 Osteogenesis of tissue engineering bone

Immune and vascularization are the key factors to regulate the osteogenesis of tissue engineering bone. Immune factors determine the inflammatory outcome and healing of the tissue. BMSCs have the ability to migrate spontaneously to the injured site and participate in the repair of corresponding tissues. BMSCs are a kind of low immunogenicity cells which can regulate the function of dendritic cells and T cells. It has the function of immune regulation and induction of immune tolerance and can improve and regulate the destructive inflammatory reaction [59, 60]. It is known that BMSCs secrete soluble factors through direct interaction between cells, inhibit the proliferation of T and B cells, inhibit the production of H_2O_2 secreted by neutrophils, and inhibit the cytotoxicity of T cells and NK cells. In vivo, BMSCs can differentiate into various tissue types when activated by various nutritional mechanisms, and the regeneration potential increases when exposed to the damaged environment. Cytokines such as IFN-α can regulate the homing and migration of BMSCs through the extracellular matrix [61]. Good vascularization can promote the supply of oxygen and nutrients, promote waste excretion, and accelerate the physiologic healing of tissue-engineered bone, which is another important factor in tissue engineering bone transplantation. Most of the tissues and cells in vivo are supplied with oxygen and nutrients by blood. Because of the limitation of oxygen diffusion in tissues, the oxygen supply range of capillaries can only be confined to the region of 100–200 μm [62]. Once implanted in vivo, the seed cells in the scaffold can only absorb oxygen

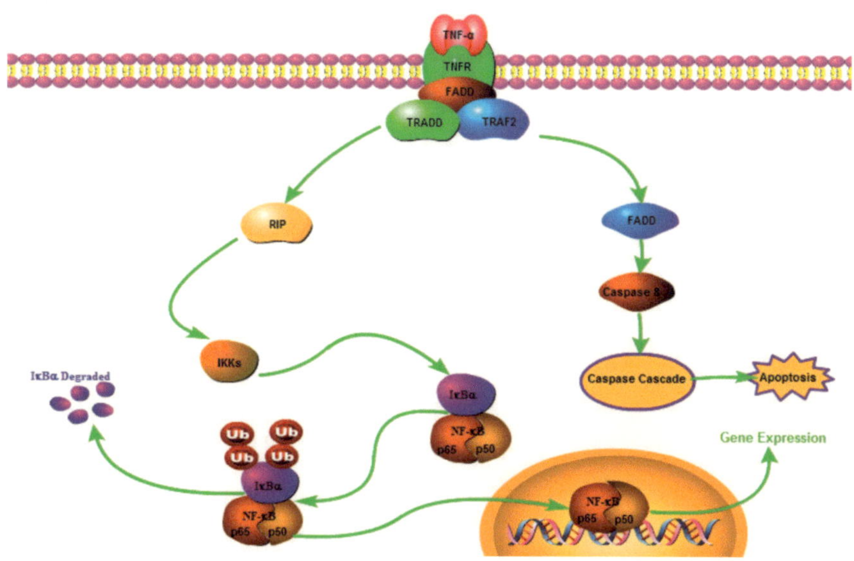

Figure 3.
TNF-α binds with TNFR1 or TNFR2 and initiates a series of signal transduction, among which FADD and NF-κB pathway determine the different destinies of the cell. The TRADD-FADD-caspase line causes apoptosis of the cell, and the TRAF2-RIP-IKKS line activates NF-κB and leads to cell survival. In fact, both routines are expressed in the cell at the same time; it is the ration of two pathways to codetermine the fate of the cell.

and nutrients through the diffusion of adjacent capillaries in the early stage. After the large tissue-engineered bone is implanted in vivo, the demand for blood supply around the scaffold is higher. The current vascularization strategies include the modification of scaffolds, the introduction of growth factors, and the combined implantation of endothelial progenitor cells. Size and roughness of materials affect immune response. Dobrovolskaia found that M1 immunoreaction was mediated when particle diameter was larger than 1 mm, and M2 immunoreaction was mediated when particle diameter was smaller than 0.5 mm [63]. Barth and other studies found that the surface roughness of materials increased, and the tendency of macrophage differentiation to M2 increased significantly, which was beneficial to promote bone regeneration [64]. Ghrebi proved that the surface roughness of biomaterials could affect the morphology of macrophages by recognizing the ERK1/ERK2 pathway activated by the adhesion protein in macrophages [65]. It is known that vascular endothelial growth factor (VEGF) [66], basic fibroblast growth factor (bFGF) [67], platelet-derived growth factor (PDGF) [67], transforming growth factor beta (TGF-β), angiopoietin l (Ang-1), and other angiogenic growth factors can promote vascularization of tissue engineering complex implanted in vivo [68]. Kim et al. encapsulated VEGF in silica nanoparticles and released them after 28 days; the study showed that this method can effectively promote angiogenesis. Endothelial progenitor cell, also known as angioblast, is involved not only in embryonic angiogenesis but also in embryonic angiogenesis [69]. Yu et al. co-cultured the endothelial progenitor cells derived from the bone marrow with osteoblasts and inoculated them on porous polycaprolactone hydroxyapatite to repair the 0.8 cm defect in the femur of rats. It was found that more capillaries and bone tissue were formed in the co-culture group than in the osteoblast group [70].

Author details

Yandong Mu[1,2]*, Lu Yang[2], Chenglong Li[2] and Wei Qing[2]

1 Department of Sichuan Academy of Medical Science and Sichuan Provincial People's Hospital, School of Medicine, University of Electronic Science and Technology, China

2 School of Medicine, University of Electronic Science and Technology, China

*Address all correspondence to: muyd@uestc.edu.cn

References

[1] Giannoni P, Mastrogiacomo M, Alini M, et al. Regeneration of large bone defects in sheep using bone marrow stromal cells. Journal of Tissue Engineering and Regenerative Medicine. 2008;**2**(5):253-262

[2] Cunniffe GM, Vinardell T, Murphy JM, et al. Porous decellularized tissue engineered hypertrophic cartilage as a scaffold for large bone defect healing. Acta Biomaterialia. 2015;**23**:82-90

[3] Dufrane D, Docquier PL, Delloye C, et al. Scaffold-free three-dimensional graft from autologous adipose-derived stem cells for large bone defect reconstruction: Clinical proof of concept. Medicine. 2015;**94**(50):e2220

[4] Park J, Yang KH. Indications and outcomes of augmentation plating with decortication and autogenous bone grafting for femoral shaft nonunions. Injury. 2013;**44**(12):1820-1825

[5] Attum B, Douleh D, Whiting PS, et al. Outcomes of distal femur nonunions treated with a combined nail/plate construct and autogenous bone grafting. Journal of Orthopaedic Trauma. 2017;**31**(9):e301-e304

[6] Li SL, Sun YQ. Autogenous femoral head bone grafting combined with total hip arthroplasty for the treatment of old dislocation of hip joint center in 16 cases. Zhongguo Gu Shang. 2015;**28**(10):924-927

[7] Melville JC, Nassari NN, Hanna IA, et al. Immediate Transoral allogeneic bone grafting for large mandibular defects. Less morbidity, more bone. A paradigm in benign tumor mandibular reconstruction? Journal of Oral and Maxillofacial Surgery. 2017;**75**(4):828-838

[8] Xu J, Sun Y, Wu T, et al. Porcine brain extract promotes osteogenic differentiation of bone marrow derived mesenchymal stem cells and bone consolidation in a rat distraction osteogenesis model. PLoS One. 2017;**12**(11):e187362

[9] Wu B, Zheng Q, Guo X, et al. Preparation and ectopic osteogenesis in vivo of scaffold based on mineralized recombinant human-like collagen loaded with synthetic BMP-2-derived peptide. Biomedical Materials. 2008;**3**(4):44111

[10] Zhang J, Dalbay MT, Luo X, et al. Topography of calcium phosphate ceramics regulates primary cilia length and TGF receptor recruitment associated with osteogenesis. Acta Biomaterialia. 2017;**57**:487-497

[11] Shadjou N, Hasanzadeh M, Khalilzadeh B. Graphene based scaffolds on bone tissue engineering. Bioengineered. 2018;**9**(1):38-47

[12] Yang Y, Zheng K, Liang R, et al. Cu-releasing bioactive glass/polycaprolactone coating on Mg with antibacterial and anticorrosive properties for bone tissue engineering. Biomedical Materials. 2017;**13**(1):15001

[13] Wu J, Zhang K, Yu X, et al. Hydration of hydrogels regulates vascularization in vivo. Biomaterials Science. 2017;**5**(11):2251-2267

[14] Allameh A, Jazayeri M, Adelipour M. In vivo vascularization of endothelial cells derived from bone marrow mesenchymal stem cells in SCID mouse model. Cell Journal. 2016;**18**(2):179-188

[15] Mattioli-Belmonte M, Teti G, Salvatore V, et al. Stem cell origin differently affects bone tissue engineering strategies. Frontiers in Physiology. 2015;**6**:266

[16] Li JH, Liu DY, Zhang FM, et al. Human dental pulp stem cell is a promising autologous seed cell for bone tissue engineering. Chinese Medical Journal. 2011;**124**(23):4022-4028

[17] Muschler GF, Nakamoto C, Griffith LG. Engineering principles of clinical cell-based tissue engineering. The Journal of Bone and Joint Surgery. American Volume. 2004;**86-A**(7):1541-1558

[18] Volkmer E, Drosse I, Otto S, et al. Hypoxia in static and dynamic 3D culture systems for tissue engineering of bone. Tissue Engineering. Part A. 2008;**14**(8):1331-1340

[19] Kanda T, Iwasaki T, Nakamura S, et al. Self-secretion of fibroblast growth factor-9 supports basal forebrain cholinergic neurons in an autocrine/ paracrine manner. Brain Research. 2000;**876**(1-2):22-30

[20] Wei F, Zhou Y, Wang J, et al. The immunomodulatory role of BMP-2 on macrophages to accelerate osteogenesis. Tissue Engineering. Part A. 2018;**24**(7-8):584-594

[21] Zhang HX, Zhang XP, Xiao GY, et al. In vitro and in vivo evaluation of calcium phosphate composite scaffolds containing BMP-VEGF loaded PLGA microspheres for the treatment of avascular necrosis of the femoral head. Materials Science & Engineering. C, Materials for Biological Applications. 2016;**60**:298-307

[22] Anderson JM, Rodriguez A, Chang DT. Foreign body reaction to biomaterials. Seminars in Immunology. 2008;**20**(2):86-100

[23] Brown BN, Badylak SF. Expanded applications, shifting paradigms and an improved understanding of host-biomaterial interactions. Acta Biomaterialia. 2013;**9**(2):4948-4955

[24] Cordova LA, Loi F, Lin TH, et al. CCL2, CCL5, and IGF-1 participate in the immunomodulation of osteogenesis during M1/M2 transition in vitro. Journal of Biomedical Materials Research. Part A. 2017;**105**(11):3069-3076

[25] Lu LY, Loi F, Nathan K, et al. Pro-inflammatory M1 macrophages promote osteogenesis by mesenchymal stem cells via the COX-2-prostaglandin E2 pathway. Journal of Orthopaedic Research. 2017;**35**(11):2378-2385

[26] Guihard P, Danger Y, Brounais B, et al. Induction of osteogenesis in mesenchymal stem cells by activated monocytes/macrophages depends on oncostatin M signaling. Stem Cells. 2012;**30**(4):762-772

[27] Loi F, Cordova LA, Zhang R, et al. The effects of immunomodulation by macrophage subsets on osteogenesis in vitro. Stem Cell Research & Therapy. 2016;**7**:15

[28] van Well G, Daalderop LA, Wolfs T, et al. Human perinatal immunity in physiological conditions and during infection. Molecular and Cellular Pediatrics. 2017;**4**(1):4

[29] Al-Maawi S, Orlowska A, Sader R, et al. In vivo cellular reactions to different biomaterials-physiological and pathological aspects and their consequences. Seminars in Immunology. 2017;**29**:49-61

[30] Kayal RA. The role of osteoimmunology in periodontal disease. BioMed Research International. 2013;**2013**:639368

[31] Kamiya N, Yamaguchi R, Adapala NS, et al. Legg-Calve-Perthes disease produces chronic hip synovitis and elevation of interleukin-6 in the synovial fluid. Journal of Bone and Mineral Research. 2015;**30**(6): 1009-1013

[32] Cafiero C, Gigante M, Brunetti G, et al. Inflammation induces osteoclast differentiation from peripheral mononuclear cells in chronic kidney disease patients: Crosstalk between the immune and bone systems. Nephrology, Dialysis, Transplantation. 2018;**33**(1):65-75

[33] Metzger CE, Narayanan A, Zawieja DC, et al. Inflammatory bowel disease in a rodent model alters osteocyte protein levels controlling bone turnover. Journal of Bone and Mineral Research. 2017;**32**(4):802-813

[34] Hoy J. Bone, fracture and frailty. Current Opinion in HIV and AIDS. 2011;**6**(4):309-314

[35] Lamba NM, Courtney JM, Gaylor JD, et al. In vitro investigation of the blood response to medical grade PVC and the effect of heparin on the blood response. Biomaterials. 2000;**21**(1):89-96

[36] Golas A, Pitakjakpipop H, Rahn MS, et al. Enzymes produced by autoactivation of blood factor XII in buffer: A contribution from the hematology at biomaterial interfaces research group. Biomaterials. 2015;**37**:1-12

[37] Hauser CJ, Otterbein LE. Danger signals from mitochondrial DAMPS in trauma and post-injury sepsis. European Journal of Trauma and Emergency Surgery. 2018;**44**(3):317-324

[38] Konrad FM, Braun S, Ngamsri KC, et al. Heme oxygenase-1 attenuates acute pulmonary inflammation by decreasing the release of segmented neutrophils from the bone marrow. American Journal of Physiology. Lung Cellular and Molecular Physiology. 2014;**307**(9):L707-L717

[39] Maderna P, Yona S, Perretti M, et al. Modulation of phagocytosis of apoptotic neutrophils by supernatant from dexamethasone-treated macrophages and annexin-derived peptide Ac(2-26). Journal of Immunology. 2005;**174**(6):3727-3733

[40] Weisser SB, McLarren KW, Kuroda E, et al. Generation and characterization of murine alternatively activated macrophages. Methods in Molecular Biology. 2013;**946**:225-239

[41] Zhou D, Huang C, Lin Z, et al. Macrophage polarization and function with emphasis on the evolving roles of coordinated regulation of cellular signaling pathways. Cellular Signalling. 2014;**26**(2):192-197

[42] Waters M, VandeVord P, Van Dyke M. Keratin biomaterials augment anti-inflammatory macrophage phenotype in vitro. Acta Biomaterialia. 2018;**66**:213-223

[43] Guo W, Imai S, Yang JL, et al. In vivo immune interactions of multipotent stromal cells underlie their long-lasting pain-relieving effect. Scientific Reports. 2017;**7**(1):10107

[44] Bing W, Pang X, Qu Q, et al. Simvastatin improves the homing of BMSCs via the PI3K/AKT/miR-9 pathway. Journal of Cellular and Molecular Medicine. 2016;**20**(5):949-961

[45] Shen X, Zhang Y, Gu Y, et al. Sequential and sustained release of SDF-1 and BMP-2 from silk fibroin-nanohydroxyapatite scaffold for the enhancement of bone regeneration. Biomaterials. 2016;**106**:205-216

[46] Chen P, Tao J, Zhu S, et al. Radially oriented collagen scaffold with SDF-1 promotes osteochondral repair by facilitating cell homing. Biomaterials. 2015;**39**:114-123

[47] Wang Y, Sun X, Lv J, et al. Stromal cell-derived factor-1 accelerates

cartilage defect repairing by recruiting bone marrow mesenchymal stem cells and promoting chondrogenic differentiation. Tissue Engineering. Part A. 2017;**23**(19-20):1160-1168

[48] Wei H, Li C, Zhao X, et al. Peripheral blood endothelial progenitor cells enhance the expressions of SDF-1 and MCP-1 of bone marrow stromal cells and promote their homing ability. Xi Bao Yu Fen Zi Mian Yi Xue Za Zhi. 2016;**32**(1):20-24

[49] Markel TA, Crafts TD, Jensen AR, et al. Human mesenchymal stromal cells decrease mortality after intestinal ischemia and reperfusion injury. The Journal of Surgical Research. 2015;**199**(1):56-66

[50] Guo Y, Wang Y, Liu Y, et al. Effect of the same mechanical loading on osteogenesis and osteoclastogenesis in vitro. Chinese Journal of Traumatology. 2015;**18**(3):150-156

[51] Kachgal S, Carrion B, Janson IA, et al. Bone marrow stromal cells stimulate an angiogenic program that requires endothelial MT1-MMP. Journal of Cellular Physiology. 2012;**227**(11):3546-3555

[52] Cassetta L, Cassol E, Poli G. Macrophage polarization in health and disease. ScientificWorldJournal. 2011;**11**:2391-2402

[53] He XT, Li X, Yin Y, et al. The effects of conditioned media generated by polarized macrophages on the cellular behaviours of bone marrow mesenchymal stem cells. Journal of Cellular and Molecular Medicine. 2018;**22**(2):1302-1315

[54] Gong D, Shi W, Yi SJ, et al. TGFbeta signaling plays a critical role in promoting alternative macrophage activation. BMC Immunology. 2012;**13**:31

[55] Arora S, Dev K, Agarwal B, et al. Macrophages: Their role, activation and polarization in pulmonary diseases. Immunobiology. 2018;**223**(4-5):383-396

[56] Mitsi E, Kamng'Ona R, Rylance J, et al. Human alveolar macrophages predominately express combined classical M1 and M2 surface markers in steady state. Respiratory Research. 2018;**19**(1):66

[57] Raggi F, Pelassa S, Pierobon D, et al. Regulation of human macrophage M1-M2 polarization balance by hypoxia and the triggering receptor expressed on myeloid cells-1. Frontiers in Immunology. 2017;**8**:1097

[58] van Putten SM, Ploeger DT, Popa ER, et al. Macrophage phenotypes in the collagen-induced foreign body reaction in rats. Acta Biomaterialia. 2013;**9**(5):6502-6510

[59] Kiernan CH, KleinJan A, Peeters M, et al. Allogeneic chondrogenically differentiated human bone marrow stromal cells do not induce dendritic cell maturation. Journal of Tissue Engineering and Regenerative Medicine. 2018;**12**(6):1530-1540

[60] Di Nicola M, Carlo-Stella C, Magni M, et al. Human bone marrow stromal cells suppress T-lymphocyte proliferation induced by cellular or nonspecific mitogenic stimuli. Blood. 2002;**99**(10):3838-3843

[61] Su Y, Cheng R, Zhang J, et al. Interferon-alpha2b gene-modified human bone marrow mesenchymal stem cells inhibit hepatocellular carcinoma by reducing the Notch1 levels. Life Sciences. 2015;**143**:18-26

[62] Carmeliet P, Jain RK. Angiogenesis in cancer and other diseases. Nature. 2000;**407**(6801):249-257

[63] Dobrovolskaia MA, McNeil SE. Immunological properties of engineered

nanomaterials. Nature Nanotechnology. 2007;**2**(8):469-478

[64] Barth KA, Waterfield JD, Brunette DM. The effect of surface roughness on RAW 264.7 macrophage phenotype. Journal of Biomedical Materials Research. Part A. 2013;**101**(9):2679-2688

[65] Ghrebi S, Hamilton DW, Douglas WJ, et al. The effect of surface topography on cell shape and early ERK1/2 signaling in macrophages; linkage with FAK and Src. Journal of Biomedical Materials Research. Part A. 2013;**101**(7):2118-2128

[66] Diana D, Di Stasi R, De Rosa L, et al. Structural investigation of the VEGF receptor interaction with a helical antagonist peptide. Journal of Peptide Science. 2013;**19**(4):214-219

[67] De Marchis F, Ribatti D, Giampietri C, et al. Platelet-derived growth factor inhibits basic fibroblast growth factor angiogenic properties in vitro and in vivo through its alpha receptor. Blood. 2002;**99**(6):2045-2053

[68] Suliman S, Sun Y, Pedersen TO, et al. In vivo host response and degradation of copolymer scaffolds functionalized with nanodiamonds and bone morphogenetic protein 2. Advanced Healthcare Materials. 2016;**5**(6):730-742

[69] Asahara T, Murohara T, Sullivan A, et al. Isolation of putative progenitor endothelial cells for angiogenesis. Science. 1997;**275**(5302):964-967

[70] Yu H, VandeVord PJ, Mao L, et al. Improved tissue-engineered bone regeneration by endothelial cell mediated vascularization. Biomaterials. 2009;**30**(4):508-517

Chapter 5

Traditional Chinese Medicine Therapy for Targeting Osteoblastogenesis

Yanqiu Liu

Abstract

Osteoblasts are derived from bone marrow mesenchymal stem cell (BMSC) precursors, which differentiate into mature osteoblasts and mediate bone formation. This process is called osteoblastogenesis. A deficiency in osteoblastogenesis of BMSCs can result in bone-related diseases including osteoporosis. Thus, developing drugs for targeting osteoblastogenesis from BMSCs has become one of the therapeutic strategies for osteoporosis. In China, kidney-nourishing Chinese herbal drugs such as ER-Zhi-Wan have been believed to be potential for treating osteoporosis through targeting osteoblast proliferation and differentiation. The key pathways for regulating osteoblastogenesis include canonical and noncanonical Wnt pathway, semaphorin-mediated pathway, and MAPK-mediated BMP2-Smad pathway. Some natural products have been confirmed to regulate more than one pathway and exert multi-target effect through the use of one compound or combined use of more than two compounds, such as wedelolactone and oleonuezhenide. In addition, tissue engineering provides a promising strategy in the field for targeting osteoblastogenesis. New types of biomaterials including hydroxyapatite (HAp) combined with Chinese medicine can exert enhanced effect on osteoblastogenesis and provide new therapy for treating osteoporosis.

Keywords: targets, osteoblastogenesis, traditional Chinese medicine, Wnt pathway, semaphorins, biomaterials

1. Introduction

The bone is a dynamic organ, capable of regenerating and remodeling throughout the lifetime. Bone remodeling is a process, which is mainly balanced by osteoblast-mediated bone formation and osteoclast-mediated bone resorption. Bone marrow mesenchymal stem cells (BMSCs) are osteoprogenitors, which differentiates into maturated osteoblasts and mediated bone formation, therefore maintaining the balance of bone remodeling. The process of osteoblast proliferation and differentiation from BMSCs is called osteoblastogenesis, which plays a key role for osteogenesis. A decrease in osteoblastogenesis of mesenchymal stem cells is observed to result in bone-related diseases, such as osteoporosis [1, 2]. Stimulation of proliferation and osteoblastogenesis from BMSCs becomes a therapeutic strategy for osteoporosis. A large number of factors have been implicated in regulating osteoblast differentiation, such as the Wnt family [3, 4]. Canonical Wnt signaling is crucial for regulation of osteoblast development including osteoblast proliferation, differentiation, and survival. Activation of the canonical Wnt signaling pathway involves recruitment of a complex including LRP5/6 and GSK3β, stabilization of β-catenin, regulation of transcription factors such as runx2, and activation of Wnt target genes [5]. This pathway is active in BMSCs, and therefore many signaling molecules are developed as drug targets such as GSK3β and LRP5/6. Noncanonical Wnt signaling pathway is mediated by Wnt5a, which activates downstream pathways including Wnt/Ca^{2+}/PKC, small GTPase Rho, and JNK pathways [6]. Consequently, transcription factors, such as AP1 family [7], are activated, and survival-related gene expression is induced. The anabolic agents, such as parathyroid hormone (PTH), are developed to treat osteoporosis through enhancing osteoblastogenesis. However, administration of PTH_{1-34} for a long time can increase bone resorption, resulting in bone neurosis [8]. Therefore, research is currently focusing on drugs that can simultaneously regulate bone resorption and bone formation and could thus develop a new class of dual-action therapeutic agents for osteoporosis [9, 10].

According to traditional Chinese medicine theory, "kidney-nourishing" herbal drugs are commonly believed to have the ability of nourishing bones and therefore are used to treat osteoporosis. Traditional Chinese herbs have the characteristics of multi-components and multi-target; thus the development of bifunctional agents from traditional Chinese herbs is promising. Many potential compounds isolated from "kidney-nourishing" herbal drugs have been found to enhance osteoblastogenesis [11]. We focus on a traditional Chinese prescription, called Er-Zhi-Wan, which consists of Ecliptae herba and *Fructus Ligustri Lucidi*. Extract of Er-Zhi-Wan has been reported to increase bone volume and enhance bone formation. We determine the components by using HPLC-MS method and screen the active compounds. Wedelolactone isolated from Ecliptae herba is firstly reported to inhibit osteoclastogenesis and simultaneously enhance osteoblastogenesis. In ovariectomized mice, administration of wedelolactone prevented ovariectomy-induced bone loss by enhancing osteoblast activity and inhibiting osteoclast activity. At the molecular level, wedelolactone altered several key signaling pathways. Wedelolactone facilitated osteoblastogenesis through activation of Wnt/GSK3β/β-catenin signaling pathway, which led to the activation of runx2 and the expression of downstream genes. Simultaneously, wedelolactone inhibited osteoclastogenesis through inhibition of RANKL/RANK/NF-κB pathway, resulting in suppression of c-Fos/NFATc1 activation and osteoclast marker gene expression. Although wedelolactone can treat osteoporosis with the characteristics of bifunctional activity, wedelolactone is not perfect. At the high dose, wedelolactone can trigger cytotoxicity against BMSCs. Therefore, we propose that components from *Fructus Ligustri Lucidi* could alleviate wedelolactone-induced cytotoxicity, since it is believed that the synergy effect contributes for the improved therapeutic efficacies.

Several compounds from *Fructus Ligustri Lucidi* are determined to have the ability to enhancing osteoblastogenesis. Among them, oleonuezhenide is found to increase bone mineralization induced by wedelolactone. Additionally, high dose of wedelolactone-induced cytotoxicity in BMSCs was relieved by addition of oleonuezhenide, and these BMSCs protected by oleonuezhenide maintained osteoblastic activity. These data further confirm that oleonuezhenide enhances wedelolactone's action on osteoblast differentiation and activity through Wnt/CK2α/β-catenin pathway and prevents wedelolactone-induced cytotoxicity through Wnt5a/CK2α/ERK pathway, indicating that combination of different compounds generates multi-target effect. This might contribute for the efficacy for the mixture of different herbal drugs.

In addition to the development of new type of drugs for targeting osteoblastogenesis, tissue engineering provides a promising strategy in the field for osteogenesis from BMSCs, which aims to induce new, BMSC-driven, bone regeneration and has increased the possibility of engineering bone in vitro to treat bone defects particularly in vivo [12]. As alternatives polymeric biomaterials are applied in clinical practice since the 1960s; their popularity is related to the ease of preparation of various products in complex shapes and a wide range of physical and mechanical properties. Hydroxyapatite (HAp) is a major mineral component of calcified tissues including bones. Synthetic HAp has been extensively used as an important material for bone substitute, owing to its excellent osteoinductive properties. However, most HAp is considered to be weak in osteoinductive ability, which may impact the repair capacity for bone defects. Thus, the combined effect of HAp, growth factors, or osteoinductive agents such as natural products on osteoblastogenesis might be promising. We investigate the action of incorporation of wedelolactone and HAp nanoparticles with different shapes and sizes on osteoblastogenesis from BMSCs. First, HAps are constructed by a rodlike shape with different particle sizes. HAp-1 combined with wedelolactone induced a higher ALP activity with different degrees, suggesting that combination of biomaterial and compounds contributes for osteoblastogenesis and thus can be used as therapeutic strategy for osteoporosis. Overall, this chapter will discuss recent findings regarding osteoblastogenesis and its related therapeutic strategies.

2. Osteoblastogenesis and its related therapies

2.1 The cellular and molecular mechanism of osteoblastogenesis

Osteoblasts arise from bone marrow mesenchymal stem cell (BMSC) precursor, which differentiates into maturated osteoblasts and mediated bone formation. The maturated osteoblasts synthesize dense, cross-linked collagen and specialized proteins in much smaller quantities, including osteocalcin and osteopontin, which compose the organic matrix of bone. This organic matrix forms a strong and dense mineralized tissue—the mineralized matrix.

Along with osteoblasts, osteoclast breaks down bone matrix. The balance of bone formation and bone resorption maintained bone homeostasis [13]. However, the balance tends to be negative with age, particularly in postmenopausal women, often leading to a loss of bone serious enough to cause fractures, which is called osteoporosis. A decrease in osteoblastogenesis of mesenchymal stem cells can be observed in osteoporosis [2]. Reduced proliferation and osteoblastic differentiation of BMSCs were reported to associate with the reduction of healing capacity such as impairment of bone formation in osteoporotic patients. Therefore, stimulation of proliferation and osteoblastogenesis from BMSCs becomes a therapeutic strategy for osteoporosis.

There are several signaling pathways involved in osteoblastogenesis. BMP (bone morphogenetic protein) signaling is a fundamental pathway that mediates osteoblast differentiation [14]. BMP signaling is mediated through type I and type II BMP receptors. After binding to BMP ligands, BMP receptors formed a complex. This dynamic interaction leads to signal transduction through either Smads or mitogen-activated protein kinases (MAPKs) which further activates the transcription of specific target genes involved in osteoblastic differentiation and bone formation [15]. Several MAPKs have been identified, including extracellular signal-regulated kinases (ERKs), c-Jun N-terminal protein kinase (JNK), and p38 MAPK. These three types of MAPKs are essential components of the signal transduction machinery that occupy central positions in this differentiation process [16]. Following activation of MAPK signaling during this differentiation process, BMP2/Smad signaling is activated.

Canonical and noncanonical Wnt signaling pathways play key roles in the regulation of osteoblast development including enhancement of osteoblast proliferation as well as differentiation [17]. The canonical Wnt/GSK3β/β-catenin signaling is a key pathway for regulating bone formation and contributing to osteoblastic differentiation. Canonical Wnt pathway involves the formation of a complex consisting of Wnt1, 3a proteins, Frizzed, LRP5/6, and GSK3β. A crucial step in transducting the Wnt signal is to destroy the cytoplasmic GSK3β complex by inducing GSK3β phosphorylation and subsequently, inhibits β-catenin phosphorylation, thereby stabilizing β-catenin. The accumulated β-catenin thus enters the nucleus and activates the expression of the Wnt target genes. These target genes include marker genes for osteoblastogenesis. Alkaline phosphatase is a membrane-anchored protein that is a characteristic marker expressed in large amounts at the apical (secretory) face of active osteoblasts. Other marker genes, including SP7 (which encodes osterix) and Bglap (encoding osteocalcin), were markedly increased in their expression during the osteogenic differentiation. Runx2 is the master osteogenic transcription factor that takes part in the process of osteoblast maturation. Runx2 is also found to transduce Wnt signaling for mediating osteogenic differentiation of BMSCs [18]. It can act as crosstalking regulator between Wnt signaling pathways and others that enhance osteoblastogenesis. The canonical Wnt signaling pathway is active in BMSCs, and therefore many signaling molecules are developed as drug targets such as GSK3β and LRP5/6.

Noncanonical Wnt signaling pathway is mediated by Wnt5a, which activates downstream pathways including Wnt/Ca^{2+}/PKC, small GTPase Rho, and JNK pathways [19]. Noncanonical Wnt signaling pathway has been reported to regulate many cellular processes, including gene expression, cell proliferation, and apoptosis. Wnt5a can interact with Fz receptor and activates the cytoplasmic protein Dvl2 through casein kinase 2α (CK2α), which induces the activation of downstream molecules such as RhoA and ERK1/2. CK2 is a key regulator both in canonical and noncanonical Wnt signaling pathways [20, 21]. CK2α is its catalytic subunit. CK2α can induce nuclear translocation of β-catenin and thereby precluding degradation mediated by the proteasome. CK2α can also induce disheveled activation and therefore acts as a switch to define distinct branches of noncanonical Wnt signaling pathways. Although CK2α was developed as targets for embryogenesis, neuronal differentiation, and myogenic differentiation, the role of CK2α for osteoblastogenesis is still unclear.

Semaphorins are a family of cell-surface or soluble proteins that are able to regulate cell-cell interactions as well as cell differentiation, morphology, and function. In the mammalian system, 20 semaphorins have been identified and fall into 5 classes (semaphorins 3–7) that are characterized by particular structural properties [22]. Among them, Sema3A play a key role in coupling of osteoblastogenesis and osteoclastogenesis. Sema3A is produced by osteoblasts and has been identified as a potent and direct inhibitor of osteoclast formation from osteoclast precursor cells. Distinct from other coupling factors, Sema3A promotes osteoblast differentiation from BMSCs (the precursor of osteoblasts), indicating a dual function role in which it inhibits osteoclastogenesis and enhances osteoblastogenesis [23]. The Sema3A signaling pathway is activated through binding with its cell-surface receptor composed of an Nrp1 and plexinA1 protein complex, which functions as a signal-transducing subunit [24]. This complex induces different downstream signaling molecules in osteoclasts and osteoblasts, resulting in different regulatory effects on differentiation. Therefore, regulation of the Sema3A pathway in osteoclasts and osteoblasts would be promising for the bone remodeling balance and be helpful for the development of therapeutic agents.

In addition to Sema3A, several other semaphorins play a role in osteogenesis. They can be expressed on osteoclast or osteoblast. Sema3A and Sema3E are produced from osteoblasts, while Sema4D and Sema6D are expressed by osteoclasts. Sema7A can be expressed in both osteoblasts and osteoclasts. The role of semaphorin family proteins in osteoblast and osteoclast is different [25–27]. Sema3E are produced from osteoblasts, while Sema4D and Sema6D are expressed by osteoclasts. Sema7A can be expressed in both osteoblasts and osteoclasts. The role of semaphorin family proteins in osteoblast and osteoclast is different. Sema7A is reported to be expressed in osteoblasts and promoted the osteoblast migration [28]. In addition to Sema7A, expression level of Sema3E from mouse osteoblasts was reported to be increased by PTH and 1, 25-(OH)2 D3 treatment [29]. The effects of semaphorins are mediated by plexins, a group of nine transmembrane receptors that can be subdivided into four classes, plexins A–D. The semaphorin-plexin system has an important role in regulating bone cell function. Therefore, regulating the balance of semaphorin family protein levels and semaphorin-mediated signaling pathway might balance bone remodeling through enhancing osteoblastogenesis and simultaneously inhibiting osteoclastogenesis.

2.2 Chinese herbal drugs for targeting osteoblastogenesis

2.2.1 Traditional Chinese medicine theory

Traditional Chinese medicine (TCM) is a style of traditional medicine built on a foundation of more than 2500 years of Chinese medical practice that includes various forms of herbal medicine, acupuncture, massage (tui na), exercise (qigong), and dietary therapy [30] but recently is also influenced by modern Western medicine.

One of the basic theories of TCM is zàng-fǔ theory. The term zàng refers to the five entities, including the heart, liver, spleen, lung, and kidney, while fǔ refers to the six yang organs, including the small intestine, large intestine, gallbladder, urinary bladder, stomach, and Sānjiaō [31]. Among them, the kidney is considered to be related to bones. As distinct from the Western medical definition of kidneys, the TCM concept is more a way of describing a set of interrelated parts than an anatomical organ. The main functions of the kidney are to strengthen bones, dominate human growth and development, produce marrow to fill up the brain, etc. (**Figure 1**).

According to the Chinese medicine kidney theory, many kidney-nourishing herbal drugs can strengthen bones; therefore they are used for treatment of bone-related diseases such as osteoporosis. Enhancement of osteoblastogenesis might be one of the mechanisms of action of these herbs. A famous Chinese doctor named

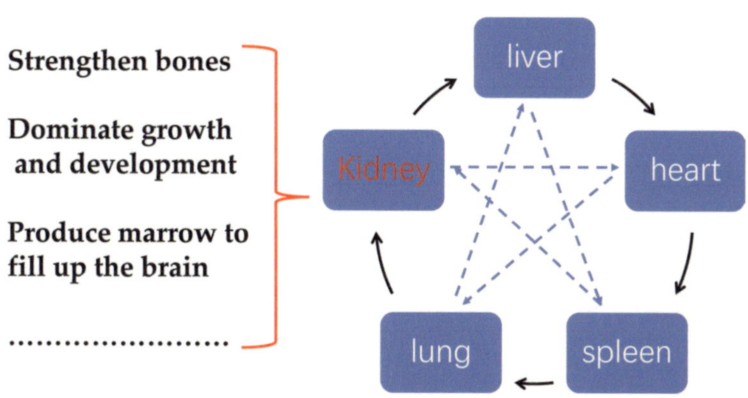

Figure 1.
The relationship of zàng-fǔ Chinese medicine theory and strengthen bones.

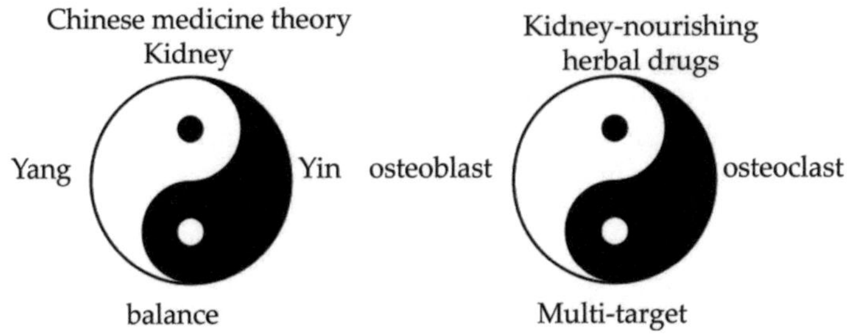

Figure 2.
Different regulated roles of kidney yin and yang in osteoblastogenesis. Kidney yang and yin might alter osteoblast and osteoclast function and enhance osteoblastogenesis and inhibiting osteoclastogenesis.

Zhang Jie Bin (approximately 1563–1640) wrote "there are two kidneys, (kidney yin and yang), with the gate of vitality between them" (**Figure 2**). The difference between kidney yin and kidney yang on strengthening bones is still unclear, but the different mechanisms of action of kidney yin and yang on osteoblastogenesis might partially explain the difference.

2.2.2 Chinese herbal drugs that enhance osteoblastogenesis and/or inhibiting osteoclastogenesis

Many kidney-tonifying herbal drugs are found to regulate osteoblastogenesis. Some are kidney-yang herbal drugs, including *Herba Epimedii*, *Taxus yunnanensis*, *Rhizoma Drynariae*, etc. Some are kidney-yin herbal drugs, including *Eclipta* herbal and *Fructus Ligustri Lucidi*. *Herba Epimedii* is a commonly used Chinese medicine as "kidney yang" herbs for thousands of years. It contains active components such as flavonoids and phytosteroids. Total flavonoids of *Herba Epimedii* are suggested to enhance osteoblast proliferation and differentiation and to be potential candidates for treating osteoporosis [32]. It includes icariin, epimedin A, epimedin B, epimedin C, icariside II, icaritin, etc. Although icariin is a principal flavonoid glycoside in *Herba Epimedii*, icariside II and icaritin, two hydrolytic metabolites in vivo as well as present in *Herba Epimedii*, showed higher activity of osteoblast proliferation and differentiation [33, 34] (**Table 1**).

Ecliptae herba, also known as "Mo-Han-Lian," is the aerial parts of *Eclipta prostrata* L. (Asteraceae), which have antiosteoporotic effect [45, 46]. Wedelolactone is a compound isolated from Ecliptae herba. Although ethyl acetate extract of Ecliptae herba and wedelolactone did not change BMSC proliferation, the extract and wedelolactone enhance BMSC differentiation toward osteoblasts. BMSC incubation with wedeloloactone results in an increase in the activity of alkaline phosphatase (ALP), a marker enzyme for maturated osteoblasts, in a dose-dependent manner. Also, mineralization level and calcium deposits increased accordingly in response to wedelolactone. At the molecular level, wedelolactone directly inhibited GSK3β activity and enhanced the phosphorylation of GSK3β and thereafter stimulated the nuclear translocation of β-catenin and runx2. The expression of osteoblastogenesis-related marker gene including osteorix, osteocalcin, and runx2 was increased. In ovariectomized mice, administration of wedelolactone prevented ovariectomy-induced bone loss by enhancing osteoblast activity and promoting new bone formation [47].

Distinct with other osteogenic agent, such as PTH_{1-34}, wedelolactone exert dual function role in enhancing osteoblastogenesis and simultaneously inhibiting osteoclastogenesis. For the anabolic agent, parathyroid hormone (PTH) a concomitant

Compounds or extracts	Herbal drugs or plants	Validation	Refs.
Icarrin, icariside II, icaritin	*Herba Epimedii*	Enhance osteoblast proliferation and differentiation	[34]
Wedelolactone	Ecliptae herba	Promote osteoblast differentiation and bone formation	[35, 36]
Specnuezhenide, ligustroflavone, salidroside, and Gl3	*Fructus Ligustrum lucidum*	Stimulate osteoblast proliferation and bone formation by BMP2 and runx2 activation	[37, 38]
Puerariae radix extract	*Puerariae radix*	Play a role in osteoblastic bone formation; induces osteoblastic differentiation markers such as ALP, OCN, OPN, and Col I and mineralization in SaOS-2 cells	[39]
Tetrahydroxystilbene glucoside	*Fallopia multiflora*	Promote osteoblast differentiation	[40]
Total flavonoids	*Rhizoma Drynariae*	Enhance osteoblast activity through BMP2/Smad pathway	[41]
Aqueous extract	*Angelica sinensis*	Stimulate proliferation and ALP activity of OPC-1	[42]
Extract	*Salvia miltiorrhiza*	Stimulates ALP activity in MC3T3-E1 cells	[43]
Extract	*Astragalus membranaceus*	Promote new bone formation on periodontal defects in vivo	[44]

Table 1.

Cellular and molecular targets for different herbal drugs with the ability of enhancing osteoblastogenesis.

increase in bone resorption can be observed. These drawbacks of the current therapies might be attributed to one target for these drugs that fail to uncouple bone degradation and formation: they stimulate or inhibit both processes at the same time. Research is currently focusing on drugs that can simultaneously regulate bone resorption and bone formation. Wedelolactone might be potential for the development of new class of drugs for treating osteoporosis. Further, the dual function of wedelolactone might be attributed to multi-target action on osteogenesis.

In addition to Wnt/GSK3β/β-catenin pathway activation by wedelolactone, we found that the semaphorin 3A pathway, as the upstream of Wnt/GSK3β/β-catenin pathway, was activated. Wedelolactone can increase mRNA expression of Sema3A in BMSCs and blocking Sema3A activity with its antibody reversed wedelolactone-induced alkaline phosphatase activity in BMSCs. Further, wedelolactone enhanced binding of Sema3A with cell-surface receptors, including neuropilin (NRP)1 and plexinA1. In addition, nuclear accumulation of β-catenin, a transcription factor acting downstream of wedelolactone-induced Sema3A signaling, was blocked by the Sema3A antibody. For the osteoclasts, a 9 day incubation fraction of conditioned media obtained from wedelolactone-treated bone marrow mesenchymal stem cell (BMSC) significantly inhibited tartrate-resistant acid phosphatase (TRAP) activity in RANKL-stimulated osteoclastic RAW264.7 cells. Conditioned media and wedelolactone promoted the formation of plexinA1-Nrp1, but conditioned media also caused these sequestration of the plexinA1-DNAX-activating protein12 (DAP12) complex and suppressed the phosphorylation of phospholipase C (PLC)γ2. These data suggest that wedelolactone promoted osteoblastogenesis through production of Sema3A, thus inducing the formation of a Sema3A-plexinA1-Nrp1 complex and β-catenin activation. In osteoclastic RAW264.7cells, wedelolactone inhibited osteoclastogenesis through sequestration of the plexinA1-DAP12 complex, induced the formation of plexinA1-Nrp1 complex, and suppressed PLCγ2 activation [48].

Semaphorin family proteins exert different roles in wedelolactone-enhance osteoblastogenesis and wedelolactone-inhibited osteoclastogenesis. In addition to Sema3A, osteogenic medium(OS)-reduced Sema7A mRNA expression and OS-enhanced Sema3E mRNA expression in BMSCs were reversed by wedelolactone, but OS-reduced Sema3B mRNA expression had no change. Although there is evidence of the role of Sema3B in bone remodeling [49], OS treatment decreased Sema3B mRNA expression. Wedelolactone and Sema3B antibody did not affect ALP activity. Sema3B is reported to inhibit the proliferation and induce apoptosis in various types of cancers. Whether Sema3B has a role in BMSC proliferation and apoptosis is needed to be further studied. Wedelolactone enhanced the binding of Sema7A with plexinC1 and Beta1, but addition of Sema7A antibody partially blocked the binding triggered by wedelolactone. At the same time, addition of Sema4D antibody to wedelolactone-treated osteoclastic RAW264.7 cells showed a more significant decrease in TRAP activity and bone resorption pit formation. Wedelolactone inhibited the production of Sema4D and formation of Sema4D-PlexinB1 complex. Overall, wedelolactone inhibited the production of Sema4D and formation of Sema4D-PlexinB1 complex in RAW264.7 cells, thereafter inhibiting osteoclastogenesis. At the same time, wedelolactone enhanced osteoblastogenesis through promoting the production of Sema7A and Sema7A-PlexinC1-Beta1 complex formation in BMSCs. These results suggested that wedelolactone enhanced osteoblastogenesis but inhibited osteoclastogenesis through altering semaphorin family proteins [50].

BMP signaling pathways have a critical role in bone-formation process, and their effects can be mediated by Smad signaling. Among BMP family proteins, BMP2 has been reported to be essential for inducing bone formation [51]. Several studies have reported that MAPK signaling including JNK, ERK, and p38 pathways are involved in osteoblastogenesis [52]. p38 MAPK is required for osteoblast differentiation and induction of osteogenic marker genes. Also, p38 activation has been observed in lactoferrin-treated MC3T3-E1 cells. However, there is evidence that osteoblast differentiation is stimulated by activation of ERK and JNK, but not by activation of p38 MAPK [53]. Wedelolactone increased phosphorylation of extracellular signal-regulated kinases (ERKs), c-Jun N-terminal protein kinase (JNK), and p38 in BMSCs. Phosphorylation of mitogen-activated protein kinases (MAPKs), ERK, and JNK started to increase on day 3 of treatment, and p38 phosphorylation was increased by day 6 of treatment. Expression of bone morphogenetic protein (BMP)2 mRNA and phosphorylation of Smad1/5/8 was enhanced after treatment of cells with wedelolactone for 6 and 9 days. The addition of the JNK inhibitor SP600125, ERK inhibitor PD98059, and p38 inhibitor SB203580 suppressed wedelolactone-induced alkaline-phosphatase activity and bone mineralization. Increased expression of BMP2 mRNA and Smad1/5/8 phosphorylation was blocked by SP600125 and PD98059, but not by SB203580. Our findings confirmed that wedelolactone enhanced osteoblastogenesis through induction of the JNK- and ERK-mediated BMP2-Smad1/5/8 pathway [54].

Wedelolactone is the derivation of coumarin, which can target estrogen receptor and exert estrogenic activity. Wedelolactone also was found to be docked onto the crystal structure of GSK3β through electrostatic or hydrophobic interactions. Therefore, wedelolactone might exert multi-target effect and induce the signaling network for enhancing osteogenesis (**Figure 3**). However, wedelolactone at high dose has cytotoxicity against BMSC survival. Also, the concentration of wedelolactone into the blood is lower, which limited the application for treatment of osteoporosis in clinic. We suppose that other components combined with wedelolactone can exert synergetic effect.

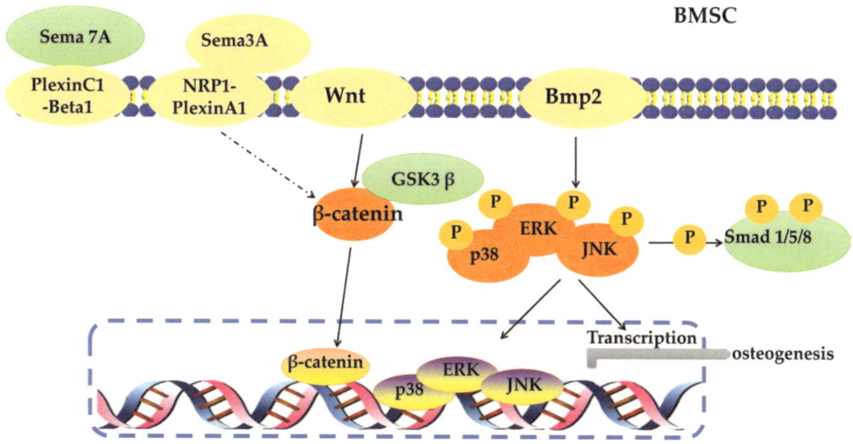

Figure 3.
Involvement of signaling network in wedelolactone-induced osteoblastogenesis. Wedelolactone induced Sema7A, 3A-mediated signaling pathway, activated downstream of β-catenin nuclear translocation, and promoted BMP2/Smad1/5/8 pathway activation, resulting in enhancement of osteoblastogenesis.

Er-Zhi-Wan is composed of Herba Ecliptae and *Fructus Ligustri Lucidi*, which is a famous traditional Chinese formulation firstly recorded in "Yi Bian" written in Ming Dynasty, which possesses the actions of tonifying the liver and kidney yin, nourishing body's essential fluid, and arresting hemorrhage. Er-Zhi-Wan extracts have been reported to prevent osteoporosis and inhibit osteoclast differentiation [55]. Er-Zhi-Wan containing serum inhibited proliferation and differentiation of preosteoclastic RAW264.7 cells. Therefore, we screened the synergetic components from *Fructus Ligustrum Lucidum*.

Fructus Ligustrum Lucidum (FLL), also known as Nu-Zhen-Zi, is the fruit of *Ligustrum lucidum* Ait., which has been used in traditional Chinese medicine for over 1000 years to nourish the liver and the kidney and thereafter strengthen the bones. In modern research, FLL is reported to possess anticancer, antidiabetic, anti-inflammatory, and heptoprotective effects. The crude FLL extract is reported to modulate the turnover of bone and the calcium balance in ovariectomized rats [56]. It also shows that ethanol extract improves calcium balance and bone metabolism in aged female rats through enhancing bone mineralization process [57]. The predominant components isolated from FLL include flavonoids, triterpenes, phenylethanoid glycosides such as salidroside, and secoiridoid glucosides such as specnuezhenide and ligustroflavone. Salidroside, specnuezhenide, and Gl3 are reported to increase osteoblast activity in osteoblast-like UMR106 cells. Aqueous extract of FLL activates ERα/β-mediated gene transcription, but the isolated compounds are inactive [58]. Salidroside is shown to promote the proliferation of BMSCs and increase the expression and secretion of stem cell factor (SCF) [59]. However, the cellular action of FLL and its compounds regulating bone metabolism is still unclear. In our study, FLL extract and five compounds from FLL were investigated to affect alkaline phosphatase (ALP) activity of bone marrow mesenchymal stem cells (BMSCs). FLL and its five components, including salidroside, specnuezhenide, nuezhenide G13, oleonuezhenide, and ligustroflavone, facilitated BMSC differentiation toward osteoblasts partially through BMP/LPR6/runx2 pathway.

Further, the combined effects of wedelolactone and various doses of compounds from *Fructus Ligustri Lucidi*, including oleonuezhenide, salidroside, and oleanolic acid, on osteoblastogenesis were evaluated. The combination of oleonuezhenide and wedelolactone was found to exert a synergistic effect on osteoblast differentiation. Wedelolactone at 6 μM and oleonuezhenide at 9 μM enhanced osteoblast differentiation and bone mineralization. The enhanced effect was more potent when bone marrow mesenchymal stem cells were treated with a combination of wedelolactone and oleonuezhenide. Osteoblastogenesis-related marker genes including osteocalcin, runx2, and osteorix were upregulated in the presence of 6 μM wedelolactone and 9 μM oleonuezhenide. At the molecular level, oleonuezhenide did not affect GSK3β phosphorylation induced by wedelolactone but elevated casein kinase 2α (CK2α) expression, resulting in β-catenin and runx2 nuclear translocation. The addition of 4,5,6,7-tetrabromo-N,N-dimethyl-1H-benzimidazol-2-amine (DMAT), a CK2α inhibitor, blocked oleonuezhenide-induced alkaline phosphatase (ALP) activity, and simultaneously suppressed β-catenin nuclear accumulation, induced by treatment with a combination of oleonuezhenide and wedelolactone. In addition, 30 μM wedelolactone-induced cytotoxicity in bone marrow mesenchymal stem cells was relieved by 9 μM oleonuezhenide. These bone marrow mesenchymal stem cells were protected by oleonuezhenide and maintained osteoblastic activity. Oleonuezhenide increased Wnt5a and CK2α expression. Wedelolactone-reduced extracellular signal-regulated kinase (ERK) phosphorylation was reversed by oleonuezhenide. However, the addition of DMAT reduced ERK phosphorylation induced by oleonuezhenide. Taken together, these data demonstrate that 10 μM oleonuezhenide enhanced the effects of 6 μM wedelolactone on osteoblastogenesis, by GSK3β- and CK2α-mediated β-catenin activation. Thus, wedelolactone-induced cytotoxicity was prevented through CK2α-mediated ERK activation. This combined effect of wedelolactone and oleonuezhenide on osteoblastogenesis may be contributed to understanding the efficiency of Er-Zhi-Wan on curing bone-related diseases, such as osteoporosis.

2.3 Combined therapy by using biomaterials and drugs

Tissue engineering provides a promising strategy in the field for osteoblastogenesis from BMSCs, which aims to induce new, BMSC-driven, bone regeneration and has increased the possibility of engineering bone in vitro to treat bone defects particularly in vivo [60–62]. As alternatives polymeric biomaterials are applied in clinical practice since the 1960s. Their popularity is related to the ease of preparation of various products in complex shapes, their moderate price, and a wide range of physical and mechanical properties. Biocomposite scaffolds are generally used for bone tissue engineering to act as a temporary matrix and provide a suitable environment for cell proliferation, differentiation, and extracellular matrix (ECM) deposition until it is restored by new natural tissue over the desired time. Various biomaterials are designed to engineer bone tissue. The bone tissue engineering scaffolds possess non-cytotoxicity, a high surface to volume ratio, abundant porosity for the transport of nutrients and regulatory factors, interconnectivity of pores for neovascularization at the site of new tissue regeneration, and osteoconductive and osteoinductive properties. Most of these material properties are satisfied by poly(L-lactic acid)-co-poly (ε-caprolactone) (PLACL), which is a copolymer of PCL and PLLA and was found to be potential synthetic polymer for bone regeneration therapy. Osteoblasts cultured on biocompatible poly(L-lactic acid)-co-poly (ε-caprolactone)-silk fibroin-hydroxyapatite-hyaluronic acid (PLACL-SF-HAp-HA) showed a significantly higher level of proliferation and increased osteogenic differentiation and mineralization [63]. Promising polymeric biomaterials however often do not fulfill the necessary requirements for the production of suitable bone implants. One of the challenges to overcome is the proliferation of cells on the implant surface [64] which could be achieved by mimicking the natural 3D bone structure with a composite of organic polymer and inorganic components.

Hydroxyapatite (HAp) is a major mineral component of calcified tissues including bones. Synthetic HAp has been extensively used as an important material for bone substitute, owing to its excellent osteoinductive properties [65]. Synthetic HAp [Ca10(PO4) 6(OH)2) has been extensively used as an implant material for bone substitute, owing to its excellent osteoinductive properties. Calcium phosphate biomaterials (HAp-TCP) with appropriate 3D geometry are able to bind and concentrate endogenous bone morphogenetic proteins in circulation, may become osteoinductive, and can be effective carriers for bone cells. Different characteristics and sizes of HAp are developed to be generally used for bone tissue engineering, which acts as a temporary matrix and provides a suitable environment for cell proliferation, differentiation, and extracellular matrix (ECM) deposition. However, HAp is considered to be weak in osteoinductive ability, which may impact the repair capacity for bone defects. Growth factors play an important role in the process of bone formation; some scaffolds have been developed as delivery carriers for growth factors and showed great bone repair ability. However, considering the high production cost and limited active period, the clinical application of exogenous growth factors is restricted. We proposed that natural products combined with HAp might have enhanced effect on osteoblastogenesis. Three kinds of HAps constructed by a rodlike shape with particle size of 25 nm (HAp-1), 37 nm (HAp-2), and 33 nm (HAp-3) did not affect BMSC survival but induced activity of alkaline phosphatase (ALP), a marker enzyme for osteoblastogenesis. The rodlike HAp might have distinct properties for osteoblast differentiation [66]. Additionally, particle size is a very important influencing factor on activity of HAp samples. The smallest particle has the best activity might be due to its easier contact of the target in the cell. The O-H groups abundantly located in the surface of HAp-1 crystal might facilitate the hydrogen bond interaction between the HAp-1 and the protein of the cell, which is in accordance with cell activity data. The structure and activity relationship analyses give us some instruction to design new HAp samples with smaller size and more hydroxyl group to improve activity.

Interestingly, the combination of HAp-1 and wedelolactone exhibited a higher and more prolong time for ALP activity, indicating that HAp-1 and wedelolactone exerted synergetic effect on ALP activity. Recent studies have demonstrated that due to the excellent specific surface area, micro-/nano-hybrid structured HAp (micro-nano HAp) granules could be applied as carriers of drug delivery systems to enhance osteogenic ability [67]. HAp-1 treatment resulted in a more significant increase in the number of ALP staining-positive BMSCs and maintained an extended time for the increased number of ALP staining-positive BMSCs. The extended time for enhanced ALP activity in the presence of HAp-1 and wedelolactone indicates that HAp-1 might have the ability of carrying wedelolactone and subsequently sustained release of wedelolactone from the HAp-1. HAp-1 combined with wedelolactone induced a higher ALP activity for a longer time than HAp-2 and HAp-3 and also increased the bone mineralization level. Osteoblastogenesis-related marker gene expression including osteorix, osteocalcin, and runx2 were increased after BMSCs were treated with HAp-1. In conclusion, HAp, which is a major mineral component of calcified tissues including bones, with different sizes generated different effects on osteoblastogenesis. HAp-1 combined with wedelolactone exerted an enhanced effect on osteoblastic differentiation, mineralization, and osteoblastogenesis-related marker gene expression, which has potential for treating osteoporosis.

3. Conclusion

Targeting osteoblastogenesis has become a promising therapeutic strategy for treatment of osteoporosis. Several pathways including canonical and noncanonical

Wnt pathway, semaphorin pathway, and BMP/Smad pathway play a critical role in regulating osteoblastogenesis. Regulating the biological network for enhancing osteoblastogenesis and simultaneously inhibiting osteoclastogenesis might develop new type of multi-target drug for treating osteoporosis. The kidney-nourishing Chinese herbal drugs have the potential since these herbs contain many components and thus exert synergetic effect. The multi-target mechanism of Er-Zhi-Wan, a prescription record since Ming Dynasty in China, is confirmed by study of combined effect of wedelolactone and oleonuezhenide. Further study of these herbs as well as screening the active components might find novel potential drugs. Further, the development of tissue engineering biomaterials and combination with Chinese herbal drugs might generate the superior therapeutic effect.

Acknowledgements

This study was supported by a grant from the National Natural Science Foundation of China (81473545), Liaoning province plans to support innovative talents in colleges and universities (LR2017050), and the State Scholarship Fund of China (201808210086).

Conflict of interest

The authors have declared that there is no conflict of interest.

Author details

Yanqiu Liu
Institute (College) of Integrative Medicine, Dalian Medical University, Dalian, China

*Address all correspondence to: yqliu@dmu.edu.cn

References

[1] Kiernan J, Davies JE, Stanford WL. Concise review: Musculoskeletal stem cells to treat age-related osteoporosis. Stem Cells Translational Medicine. 2017;**6**:1930-1939. DOI: 10.1002/sctm.17-0054

[2] Mostafavinia A, Dehdehi L, Ghoreishi SK, Hajihossainlou B, Bayat M. Effect of in vivo low-level laser therapy on bone marrow-derived mesenchymal stem cells in ovariectomy-induced osteoporosis of rats. Journal of Photochemistry and Photobiology B: Biology. 2017;**175**:29-36. DOI: 10.1016/j.jphotobiol.2017.08.021

[3] Krishnan V, Bryant HU, Macdougald OA. Regulation of bone mass by Wnt signaling. Journal of Clinical Investigation. 2006;**116**:1202-1209. DOI: 10.1016/j.cellimm.2017.05.003

[4] Takada I, Kouzmenko AP, Kato S. Wnt and PPARc signaling in osteoblastogenesis and adipogenesis. Nature Reviews Rheumatology. 2009;**5**:442-447. DOI: 10.1038/nrrheum.2009.137

[5] Holmen SL et al. Essential role of beta-catenin in postnatal bone acquisition. Biological Chemistry. 2005;**280**:21162-21168. DOI: 10.1074/jbc.M501900200

[6] Masanori O, Nobuyuki U, Shunsuke U, Kazuhiro M, Teruhito Y, Yuko N. et alNoncanonical Wnt5a enhances Wnt/β-catenin signaling during osteoblastogenesis. Scientific Reports. 2014;**4**:1-8. DOI: 10.1038/srep04493

[7] Mohammad A. AP1 dependent transcriptional regulation in normal and leukemic hematopoiesis. Experimental Hematology. 2017;**53**:S132. DOI: 10.1016/j.exphem

[8] Cappuzzo KA, Delafuente JC. Teriparatide for severe osteoporosis. The Annals of Pharmacotherapy. 2004;**38**:294-302. DOI: 10.1345/aph.1D353

[9] Deal C. Potential new drug targets for osteoporosis. Nature Clinical Practice. Rheumatology. 2009;**5**:20-27. DOI: 10.1038/ncprheum0977

[10] Baron R. Osteoporosis therapy-dawn of the post-bisphosphonate era. Nature Reviews. Endocrinology. 2011;**8**:76-78. DOI: 10.1038/nrendo.2011.207

[11] Wang X-Q, Zou X-R, Zhang YC. From "kidneys govern bones" to chronic kidney disease, diabetes mellitus, and metabolic bone disorder: A crosstalk between traditional Chinese medicine and modern science. Evidence-based Complementary and Alternative Medicine. 2016;**2016**:4370263. DOI: 10.1155/2016/4370263

[12] Weir MD, Xu HH. Osteoblastic induction on calcium phosphate cement-chitosan constructs for bone tissue engineering. Journal of Biomedical Materials Research Part A. 2010;**94**:223-233. DOI: 10.1002/jbm.a.32665

[13] Pederson L, Ruan M, Westendorf JJ, Khosla S, Oursler MJ. Regulation of bone formation by osteoclasts involves Wnt/BMP signaling and the chemokine sphingosine-1-phosphate. Proceedings of the National Academy of Sciences of the United States of America. 2009;**105**:20764-20769. DOI: 10.1073/pnas.0805133106

[14] Daigang L, Jining Q, Jinlai L, Pengfei W, Chuan S, Liangku H, et al. LPS-stimulated inflammation inhibits BMP-9-induced osteoblastic differentiation through crosstalk between BMP/MAPK and Smad signaling. Experimental Cell Research. 2016;**341**:54-60. DOI: 10.1016/j.yexcr.2016.01.009

[15] Kakita A, Suzuki A, Ono Y, Miura Y, Itoh M, Oiso Y. Possible involvement of p38 MAP kinase in prostaglandin E1-induced ALP activity in osteoblast-like cells. Prostaglandins, Leukotrienes, and Essential Fatty Acids. 2004;**70**:469-474. DOI: 10.1016/j.plefa.2003.09.003

[16] Fu L, Tang T, Miao Y, Zhang S, Qu Z, Dai K. Stimulation of osteogenic differentiation and inhibition of adipogenic differentiation in bone marrow stromal cells by alendronate via ERK and JNK activation. Bone. 2008;**43**:40-47. DOI: 10.1016/j.bone.2008.03.008

[17] Lerner UH, Ohlsson C. The WNT system: Background and its role in bone. Journal of Internal Medicine. 2015;**277**(6):630-649. DOI: 10.1111/join.12368

[18] Nishio Y et al. Runx2-mediated regulation of the zinc finger Osterix/Sp7 gene. Gene. 2006;**372**:62-70. DOI: 10.1016/j.gene.2005.12.022

[19] Maracci C, Rodnina MV. Translational GTPases. Biopolymers. 2016;**105**:463-475. DOI: 10.1002/bip.22832

[20] Lisberg A, Ellis R, Nicholson K, Moku P, Swarup A, Dhurjati P, et al. Mathematical modeling of the effects of CK2.3 on mineralization in osteoporotic bone. CPT: Pharmacometrics & Systems Pharmacology. 2017;**8**:208-215. DOI: 10.1002/psp4.12154

[21] Bek S, Kemler R. Protein kinase CKII regulates the interaction of beta-catenin with alpha-catenin and its protein stability. Journal of Cell Science. 2002;**115**:4743-4753. DOI: 10.10.1242/jcs.00154

[22] Worzfeld T, Offermanns S. Semaphorins and plexins as therapeutic targets. Nature Reviews. Drug Discovery. 2014;**13**:603-621. DOI: 10.1038/nrd4337

[23] Hayashi M, Nakashima T, Taniguchi M, Kodama T, Kumanogoh A, Takayanagi H. Osteoprotection by semaphorin3A. Nature. 2012;**485**:69-76. DOI: 10.1038/nature11000

[24] Kang S, Kumanogoh A. Semaphorins in bone development, homeostasis, and disease. Seminars in Cell & Developmental Biology. 2013;**24**:163-171. DOI: 10.1016/j.semcdb.2012.09.008

[25] Negishi-Koga T, Takayanagi H. Bone cell communication factors and Semaphorins. BoneKEy Reports. 2012;**1**:183. DOI: 10.1038/bonekey.2012.183

[26] Negishi-Koga T, Shinohara M, Komatsu N, Bito H, Kodama T, Friedel RH, et al. Suppression of bone formation by osteoclastic expression of semaphorin 4D. Nature Medicine. 2011;**17**:1473-1480. DOI: 10.1038/nm.2489

[27] Pasterkamp RJ, Peschon JJ, Spriggs MK, et al. Semaphorin 7A promotes axon outgrowth through integrins and MAPKs. Nature. 2003;**424**:398-405. DOI: 10.1038/nature01790

[28] Delorme G, Saltel F, Bonnelye E, et al. Expression and function of semaphorin 7A in bone cells. Biology of the Cell. 2005;**97**:589-597. DOI: 10.1042/BC20040103

[29] Hughes A, Kleine-Albers J, Helfrich MH, et al. A class III semaphorin (Sema3e) inhibits mouse osteoblast migration and decreases osteoclast formation in vitro. Calcified Tissue International. 2012;**90**:151-162. DOI: 10.1007/s00223-011-9560-7

[30] Sheng X, Zhang H, Weng Q. Traditional Chinese medicine: China's bear farms prompt public outcry. Nature. 2012;**484**:455. DOI: 10.1038/484455c

[31] Matuk C. Seeing the body: The divergence of ancient Chinese and

western medical illustration. Journal of Biocommunication. 2006;**32**:1-8

[32] Zhang JF, Li G, Meng CL, Dong Q, Chan CY, He ML, et al. Total flavonoids of *Herba Epimedii* improves osteogenesis and inhibits osteoclastogenesis of human mesenchymal stem cells. Phytomedicine. 2009;**16**:521-529. DOI: 10.1016/j.phymed.2009.01.003

[33] Huang J, Yuan L, Wang X, Zhang TL, Wang K. Icaritin and its glycosides enhance osteoblastic, but suppress osteoclastic, differentiation and activity in vitro. Life Sciences. 2007;**81**:832-840. DOI: 10.1016/j.lfs.2007.07.015

[34] Liu YQ, Yang QX, Cheng MC, Xiao HB. Synergistic inhibitory effect of icariside II with icaritin from *Herba Epimedii* on pre-osteoclastic RAW264.7 cell growth. Phytomedicine. 2014;**21**:1633-1637. DOI: 10.1016/j.phymed.2014.07.016

[35] Liu YQ, Zhan LB, Liu T, Cheng MC, Liu XY, Xiao HB. Inhibitory effect of Ecliptae herba extract and its component wedelolactone on pre-osteoclastic proliferation and differentiation. Journal of Ethnopharmacology. 2014;**157**:206-211. DOI: 10.1016/j.jep.2014.09.033

[36] Lee MK, Ha NR, Yang H, Sung SH, Kim YC. Stimulatory constituents of *Eclipta prostrate* on mouse osteoblast differentiation. Phytotherapy Research. 2009;**23**:129-131. DOI: 10.1002/ptr.2560

[37] Tang Y-q, Li C, Sun X-j, Liu Y, Wang X-t, Guo Y-b, et al. *Fructus Ligustri Lucidi* modulates estrogen receptor expression with no uterotrophic effect in ovariectomized rats. BMC Complementary and Alternative Medicine. 2018;**18**:118. DOI: 10.1186/s12906-018-2171-3

[38] Wang L, Ma R, Guo Y, Sun J, Liu H, Zhu R, et al. Antioxidant effect of fructus ligustri lucidi aqueous extract in ovariectomized rats is mediated through Nox4-ROS-NF-κB pathway. Frontiers in Pharmacology. 2017;**8**:266. DOI: 10.3389/fphar.2017.00266

[39] Huh JE, Yang HR, Park DS, Choi DY, Baek YH, Cho EM, et al. *Puerariae radix* promotes differentiation and mineralization in human osteoblast-like SaOS-2 cells. Journal of Ethnopharmacology. 2006;**104**:345-350. DOI: 10.1016/0168-9002(96)00006-X

[40] Fan YS, Li Q, Hamdan N, Bian YF, Zhuang S, Fan K, et al. Tetrahydroxystilbene glucoside regulates proliferation, differentiation, and OPG/RANKL/M-CSF expression in MC3T3-E1 cells via the PI3K/Akt pathway. Molecules. 2018;**23**:E2306. DOI: 10.3390/molecules23092306

[41] Chen LL, Lei LH, Ding PH, Tang Q, Wu YM. Osteogenic effect of *Drynariae* rhizoma extracts and naringin on MC3T3-E1 cells and an induced rat alveolar bone resorption model. Archives of Oral Biology. 2011;**56**:1655-1662. DOI: 10.1016/j.archoralbio.2011.06.008

[42] Yang Q, Populo SM, Zhang J, Yang G, Kodama H. Effect of *Angelica sinensis* on the proliferation of human bone cells. Clinica Chimica Acta. 2002;**324**:89-97. DOI: 10.1016/S0009-8981(02)00210-3

[43] Wenden A, Yang Y, Chai L, Wong RW. Salvia miltiorrhiza induces VEGF expression and regulates expression of VEGF receptors in osteoblastic cells. Phytotherapy Research. 2014;**28**:673-677. DOI: 10.1002/ptr.5031

[44] Yang F, Yan G, Li Y, Han Z, Zhang L, Chen S, et al. Astragalus polysaccharide attenuated iron overload-induced dysfunction of mesenchymal stem cells via suppressing mitochondrial ROS. Cellular Physiology and Biochemistry. 2016;**39**:1369-1379. DOI: 10.1159/000447841

[45] Zhang ZG, Bai D, Liu MJ, Li Y, Pan JH, Liu H, et al. Therapeutic effect of aqueous extract from Ecliptae herba on bone metabolism of ovariectomized rats. Menopause. 2013;**20**:232-240. DOI: 10.1097/gme.0b013e318265e7dd

[46] Zhang H, Xing WW, Li YS, Zhu Z, Wu JZ, Zhang QY, et al. Effect of a traditional Chinese herbal preparation on osteoblasts and osteoclasts. Maturitas. 2009;**61**:334-339. DOI: 10.1016/j.maturitas.2008.09.023

[47] Liu YQ, Hong ZL, Zhan LB, Chu HY, Zhang XZ, Li GH. Wedelolactone enhances osteoblastogenesis by regulating Wnt/β-catenin signaling pathway but suppresses osteoclastogenesis by NF-κB/c-fos/NFATc1 pathway. Scientific Reports. 2016;**6**:32260. DOI: 10.1038/srep32260

[48] Liu YQ, Han XF, Bo JX, Ma HP. Wedelolactone enhances osteoblastogenesis but inhibits osteoclastogenesis through Sema3A/NRP1/PlexinA1 pathway. Frontiers in Pharmacology. 2016;**7**:375. DOI: 10.3389/fphar.2016.00375

[49] Sutton A, Zhang X, Dowd DR, et al. Semaphorin 3B is a 1,25-dihydroxyvitamin D3-induced gene in osteoblasts that promotes osteoclastogenesis and induces osteopenia in mice. Molecular Endocrinology. 2008;**22**:1370-1381. DOI: 10.1210/me.2007-0363

[50] Deng X, Liang LN, Zhu D, Zheng LP, Yu JH, Meng XL, et al. Wedelolactone inhibits osteoclastogenesis but enhances osteoblastogenesis through altering different semaphorins production. International Immunopharmacology. 2018;**60**:41-49. DOI: 10.1016/j.intimp.2018.04.037

[51] Huang RL, Yuan Y, Tu J, Zou GM, Li Q. Opposing TNF-α/IL-1β- and BMP-2-activated MAPK signaling pathways converge on Runx2 to regulate BMP-2-induced osteoblastic differentiation. Cell Death & Disease. 2014;**5**:e1187. DOI: 10.1038/cddis.2014.101

[52] Hata K, Ikebe K, Wada M, Nokubi T. Osteoblast response to titanium regulates transcriptional activity of Runx2 through MAPK pathway. Journal of Biomedical Materials Research Part A. 2007;**81**:446-452. DOI: 10.1002/jbm.a.31086

[53] Kim BS, Kang HJ, Park JY, Lee J. Fucoidan promotes osteoblast differentiation via JNK- and ERK-dependent BMP2-Smad 1/5/8 signaling in human mesenchymal stem cells. Experimental & Molecular Medicine. 2015;**47**:e128. DOI: 10.1038/emm.2014.95

[54] Zhu D, Deng X, Han XF, Sun XX, Pan TW, Zheng LP, et al. Wedelolactone enhances osteoblastogenesis through ERK- and JNK-mediated BMP2 expression and Smad/1/5/8 phosphorylation. Molecules. 2018;**23**:561. DOI: 10.3390/molecules23030561

[55] Cheng M, Wang Q, Fan Y, Liu X, Wang L, Xie R, et al. A traditional Chinese herbal preparation Er-Zhi-Wan, prevent ovariectomy-induced osteoporosis in rats. Journal of Ethnopharmacology. 2011;**138**:279-285. DOI: 10.1016/j/jep.2011.09.030

[56] Zhang H, Xing WW, Li YS, Zhu Z, Wu JZ, Zhang QY, et al. Effects of *Fructus Ligustri Lucidi* extract on bone turnover and calcium balance in ovariectomized rats. Biological & Pharmaceutical Bulletin. 2006;**29**:291-296. DOI: 10.1248/bpb.29.291

[57] Pang Z, Zhou ZY, Wang W, Ma Y, Niu FJ, Zhang X, et al. The advances in research on the pharmacological effects of F*ructus Ligustri Lucidi*. BioMed Research

International. 2015;**2015**:281873. DOI: 10.1155/2015/281873

[58] Chen Q, Yang L, Zhang G, Wang F. Bioactivity-guided isolation of antiosteoporotic compounds from *Ligustrum lucidum*. Phytotherapy Research. 2013;**27**:973-979. DOI: 10.1002/ptr.4820

[59] Bai H, Wang CB, Ma XH, Wei YP, Xi R, Zhao Q, et al. Effects of salidroside on proliferation of bone marrow mesenchymal stem cells. Zhongguo Shi Yan Xue Ye Xue Za Zhi. 2014;**22**:1072-1077. DOI: 10.7534/j.issn.1009-2137.2014.04.035

[60] Ha SW, Jang HL, Nam KT, Beck GR. Nano-hydroxyapatite modulates osteoblast lineage commitment by stimulation of DNA methylation and regulation of gene expression. Biomaterials. 2015;**65**:32-42. DOI: 10.1016/j.biomaterials.2015.06.039

[61] Pilloni A, Pompa G, Saccucci M, Di Carlo G, Rimondini L, Brama M, et al. Analysis of human alveolar osteoblast behavior on a nano-hydroxyapatite substrate: An in vitro study. BMC Oral Health. 2014;**14**:22. DOI: 10.1186/1472-6831-14-22

[62] Laschke MW, Witt K, Pohlemann T, Menger MD. Injectable nanocrystalline hydroxyapatite paste for bone substitution: In vivo analysis of biocompatibility and vascularization. Journal of Biomedical Materials Research. Part B, Applied Biomaterials. 2007;**82**:494-505. DOI: 10.1002/jbm.b.30755

[63] Rameshbabu N, Rao KP, Kumar TS. Accelerated microwave processing of nano-crystalline hydroxyapatite. Journal of Materials Science. 2005;**40**:6319-6323. DOI: 10.1007/s10853-005-2957-9

[64] Prakasam M, Locs J, Salma-Ancane K, Loca D, Largeteau A, Fabrication B-CL. Properties and applications of dense hydroxyapatite: A review. Journal of Functional Biomaterials. 2015;**6**:1099-1140. DOI: 10.3390/jb6041099

[65] Sujana A, Venugopal JR, Velmurugan B, Góra A, Salla M, Ramakrishna S. Hydroxyapatite-intertwined hybrid nanofibres for the mineralization of osteoblasts. Journal of Tissue Engineering and Regenerative Medicine. 2017;**11**:1853-1864. DOI: 10.1002/term.2083

[66] Sarker A, Amirian J, Min YK, Lee BT. HAp granules encapsulated oxidized alginate-gelatin-biphasic calcium phosphate hydrogel for bone regeneration. International Journal of Biological Macromolecules. 2015;**81**:898-911. DOI: 10.1016/j.ijbiomac.2015.09.029

[67] Wang G, Qiu J, Zheng L, Ren N, Li J, Liu H, et al. Sustained delivery of BMP-2 enhanced osteoblastic differentiation of BMSCs based on surface hydroxyapatite nanostructure in chitosan-HAp scaffold. Journal of Biomaterials Science, Polymer Edition. 2014;**25**:1813-1827. DOI: 10.1080/09205063.2014.951244

Chapter 6

Alternative Strategies for Stem Cell Osteogenic Differentiation

Carla Cristina Gomes Pinheiro and Daniela Franco Bueno

Abstract

Discovering strategies that increase the osteogenic differentiation potential of mesenchymal stem cells (MSCs) can lead to new perspectives for bone disease treatments. The possibility to associate the mesenchymal stem cells with scaffolds and to use them in bone regeneration as well as the number of studies to understand the signaling pathway of osteogenesis are increasing. Identifying osteogenic induction factors is extremely important and crucial for the success of bone regeneration. Studies have shown that proteins, such as bone morphogenetic proteins (BMPs), trichostatin A and IGF-1, can be efficiently used for osteogenic regeneration. However, the use of these proteins increases the treatment cost. Fortunately, low-level laser therapy (LLLT) may be a new alternative for adjuvant therapy to treat bone regeneration because it has biostimulatory effects on the conversion of mesenchymal stem cells into osteoblasts and on the induction of ex vivo ossification. The principle of tissue photobiomodulation with LLLT was first described in dermatology for healing wounds; however, other applications have been described, with anti-inflammatory and anti-edema effects and cellular proliferation and differentiation. Following this way, we will discuss some alternative strategies for osteogenic differentiation and suggest that the low-power lasers can be an innovative instrument for cell differentiation.

Keywords: osteogenesis, mesenchymal stem cells, low-level laser therapy, low-power laser, osteogenic differentiation

1. Introduction

Bone transplantation is one of the most common tissue transplants in the world, second only to blood transplant. There are approximately 15 million bone fractures per year worldwide and about 10% of those will experience no tissue regeneration, potentially leading to complications such as infections and pain [1]. Technological advances and increase in life expectancy of the global population have sparked interest in and use of alternative strategies in regenerative medicine.

Tissue bioengineering is an interdisciplinary field where engineering and biological science strategies are applied jointly in order to develop biological substitutes to restore, maintain, and/or increase the function of damaged tissues [2, 3].

In concern to bone tissue engineering different medical areas as well as dentistry areas have developed bone tissue engineering strategies (stem cells (SCs), biomaterials, and growth factors) to rehabilitate congenital malformations and craniofacial syndromes associated with bioengineering [3, 4]. Therefore, the main

IntechOpen

goal of bioengineering is to overcome limitations imposed by current conventional treatments, which are based on reconstructive surgery or organ transplant. Above all, it aims at being able to produce substitutes for organs and tissues with immune tolerance, so that transplantation can be achieved without the risk of rejection by the organism [5].

Three elements are necessary for bone tissue bioengineering: osteoconduction, osteoinduction, and osteogenesis; together, these three elements form the basis for obtaining a new, functional bone tissue [6, 7]. Given the increase in regenerative medicine studies and the need to find a biological source to promote tissue formation, that is, osteogenesis, stem cells appear to be a potentially unlimited biological source [8].

Stem cells (SCs) can be defined as cells that are capable of: (1) proliferation and self-renewal and (2) answering to external stimuli and giving rise to different specialized cell lines. Consequently, they are considered important for regenerative medicine [8]. Stem cells are classified based on their source and plasticity; hence, they can be divided into three different groups: embryonic stem cells, induced pluripotent stem cells (iPSCs), and adult stem cells.

Embryonic stem cells are those derived from the inner mass of a blastocyst (4 or 5 days after the egg has been fertilized), that are capable of differentiating in the three germ layers (endoderm, ectoderm, and mesoderm). They are known as being pluripotent. However, the therapeutic use of these cells has been questioned by several studies due to teratoma formation after transplantation in animals, potential immune rejection by the host, and strong association with ethical issues [9].

An increasing number of studies have been published about induced pluripotent stem cells (iPSCs). iPSCs are somatic cells—able to differentiate into the same cell type—but genetically altered, with four genes being inserted into their genome: OCT-4, SOX2, c-Myc, and KLF4. This increases their ability to differentiate and decreases their plasticity, changing them from somatic to pluripotent cells [9].

Another type of stem cell is the multipotent stem cell, which includes adult stem cells. They have lower plasticity than pluripotent cells and, although they can differentiate into some types of cells of adult tissues, they are unable to differentiate into germ layers. Adult stem cells are found in the body and are responsible for tissue maintenance and repair [5].

The first adult SCs described in the literature were those found in bone marrow, which have been used in the treatment of several diseases affecting the hematopoietic SCs since the 1950s. Hematopoietic SCs found in bone marrow can give rise to all types of blood cells (lymphocytes, red blood cells, platelets, etc.). In addition, studies about bone marrow transplant have led to the discovery of another important cell type—larger and adherent—that support regeneration of other tissues: the mesenchymal stem cells. Since then, several studies have begun using particularly these stem cells [10, 11].

2. Mesenchymal stem cells (MSCs)

Even after birth and growth, we can still find stem cell niches in different tissues—bone marrow, adipose tissue, skeletal muscle, dental pulp, placenta and umbilical cord, and fallopian tube—usually involved in tissue maintenance and repair [12–17].

Those are known as adult mesenchymal stem cells (MSCs). Their own characteristics are preserved, that is, they remain multipotent and undifferentiated, capable of self-renewal and differentiation into multiple cell lines—under specific in vitro conditions—including osteogenic, chondrogenic, adipogenic, and myogenic lineages [18].

The first three sources are considered key differentiation lineages in determining MSCs' multipotentiality [19]. In 1976, Friedenstein et al. isolated cells with morphological features that were described as colony-forming unit-fibroblasts (CFU-Fs). Bone marrow stromal cells were first described as bone progenitor cells present in its stromal fraction [12]. In 1991, Caplan named those stromal cells as mesenchymal stem cells with potential for cell expansion while remaining undifferentiated, the cells being a great option in cell therapy for tissue regeneration [11]. Subsequent studies have shown that these cells are able to remain undifferentiated when cultured for prolonged periods of time. Moreover, they have the ability to differentiate into mesodermal cell lineages, including chondrocytes, osteoblasts, adipocytes, and myoblasts [5].

Currently, the definition of MSCs includes several morphological and immunophenotypic factors as well as functional features. According to the International Society for Cellular Therapy (ISCT), MSCs: (i) are plastic-adherent when maintained in in vitro conditions; (ii) show positive expression of the CD13, CD29, CD44, CD54, CD73, CD90, CD105, CD166, and Stro-1 cell surface markers and negative expression of the CD14, CD19, CD34, CD45, and HLA-DR markers; and (iii) are a group of clonogenic cells, capable of differentiating into several mesodermal cell lineages [19].

A range of studies have shown that multipotent MSCs can also differentiate into unrelated germline cells in a process known as transdifferentiation. Thus, in addition to differentiating into mesodermal cells—such as bone, fat, and cartilage—MSCs also have the potential for endodermal and neuroectodermal differentiation [20]. Even though adult MSCs are generally considered to originate from mesoderm, some authors describe embryonic MSCs derived from neuroepithelium and the neural crest, such as MSCs from deciduous dental pulp [20, 21].

Adult MSCs can be isolated from several tissues, with similar membrane receptor functions and expressions. However, none of those membrane receptors is considered a MSC-specific cell surface marker; rather, MSCs show a profile of cell surface markers, with positive and negative expression, varying according to source and cell heterogeneity [22, 23].

Furthermore, important features of MSCs for clinical use are their non-immunogenicity, as described in the literature, and immunomodulatory properties, which can be observed from two different perspectives, namely: (i) immunosuppressive effects of allogeneic MSCs, inducing immune tolerance; and (ii) effect of inflammatory cytokines in MSCs' activity and differentiation, in cell-to-cell interactions [8, 24–27].

Bone marrow is considered one of the main sources of MSCs, both in experimental studies and clinical use [26]. Yet, bone marrow MSCs are obtained through a painful surgical incision that produces a low number of harvested cells [28], with only about 0.001–0.01% of the total population of nucleated cells being identified as MSCs [5, 29].

Therefore, due to the aforementioned difficulties, alternative sources of MSCs—such as lipoaspirated adipose tissue, dental pulp, umbilical cord tissue, and skeletal muscle among others—have been studied, as they are often discarded and can be easily procured and manipulated in order to obtain MSCs [16, 22, 30, 31]. Cells obtained from sources other than the bone marrow contribute greatly to the development of cell therapies and consequently to the choice of the best cellular source for clinical uses and better response to target tissue regeneration [6, 16, 17, 25].

The possibility to use a non-invasive source of MSCs in bone tissue engineering has been increased by researches, because of the ease of obtaining the tissue, since they are discarded and do not involve ethical controversy. Since the year 2000, described by Gronthos, mesenchymal stem cells derived from dental pulp (DPSCs) have been studied by other researchers, and the use of DPSCs in vitro and in vivo has generated a great expectation for the translational use in tissue bioengineering, especially for bone neoformation [8, 30–32]. The profile of DPSCs when compared to stem cells derived from human adipose tissue (hASCs), the DPSCs present an increase in the extracellular matrix formation capacity and presented expression profile for osteogenic genes (RUNX2, BGLAP and ALP) [33]. These comparative results between alternative sources for translational use may help us find the best source of stem cells for each type of tissue to being repaired.

Recently re-emerged as an attractive source of osteogenic progenitor cells (OCPs), the periosteum can be isolated from several locations in the body, such as the anterior tibia, and the spinous process [34]. Periosteal OCPs were involved in bone repair and may also differentiate in response to paracrine signals from mechanically stimulated osteocytes. However, the interconnection of load stimulation with the molecular mechanisms is still unclear. On the other hand, another group of researchers recently described the presence of an immature cell with clonal multipotency and self-renewal characteristics in the long bones and calvarium of mice denominated with periosteal stem cells (PSCs) that are also involved in the support of the bone tissue repair [35]. With the advancement of technology, a new cellular and molecular markers can be innovative therapeutic target to open the best possibilities for promising therapies.

3. Strategies for osteogenic differentiation

A basic premise for a cell to be characterized as MSC is its ability to differentiate into a range of mesenchymal tissues—as mentioned above. Thus, stimulus for osteogenic differentiation must be efficient, resulting in viable and functional cells that produce bone extracellular matrix. This functionality is highly important for cellular characterization and applications in regenerative medicine [36].

In accordance with the basic requirements for carrying out tissue bioengineering, selection and strategy of signs of differentiation (osteoinduction) are other key aspects that should be explored. These are external inducers that promote cell proliferation and differentiation to regenerate the new tissue [36–38].

The biomaterial is not only involved as a structural support but can also be used as an inducer of osteogenic factors depending on its composition. The biomaterial classes most cited in the literature are the active ceramics, biodegradable polymers, and biodegradable metals. The mechanisms of the interaction between the cell and the biomaterial as well as of the osteogenic stimuli have not been clarified yet [39].

Another growing trend in bioengineering is the use of three-dimensional (3D) culture system, this possibility of cell culture is innovative and being explored by researchers, one of the factors that draws attention to this technique is the release of bioincomparable or non-absorbable compounds and the possible customization of the area to be regenerated [40].

Osteogenic induction and differentiation are often achieved via growth factors, which—through molecular mechanisms involving pathways, such as Wnt, BMP, FGF, and PTH, and genes that are essential for osteogenesis [41], such as RUNX 2, COL, ALP, OCN, OP, BGLAP, and SSP1—play a key role in osteogenesis and osteogenic differentiation, as shown in **Figure 1** [42–44]. In this context, identifying those factors is crucial for successful tissue regeneration.

3.1 Bone morphogenetic protein (BMP)

Bone morphogenetic proteins (BMPs) are cytokines from the beta family and are used in clinical applications to stimulate bone regeneration [45]. These proteins are involved in the development of the embryo and in skeletal formation.

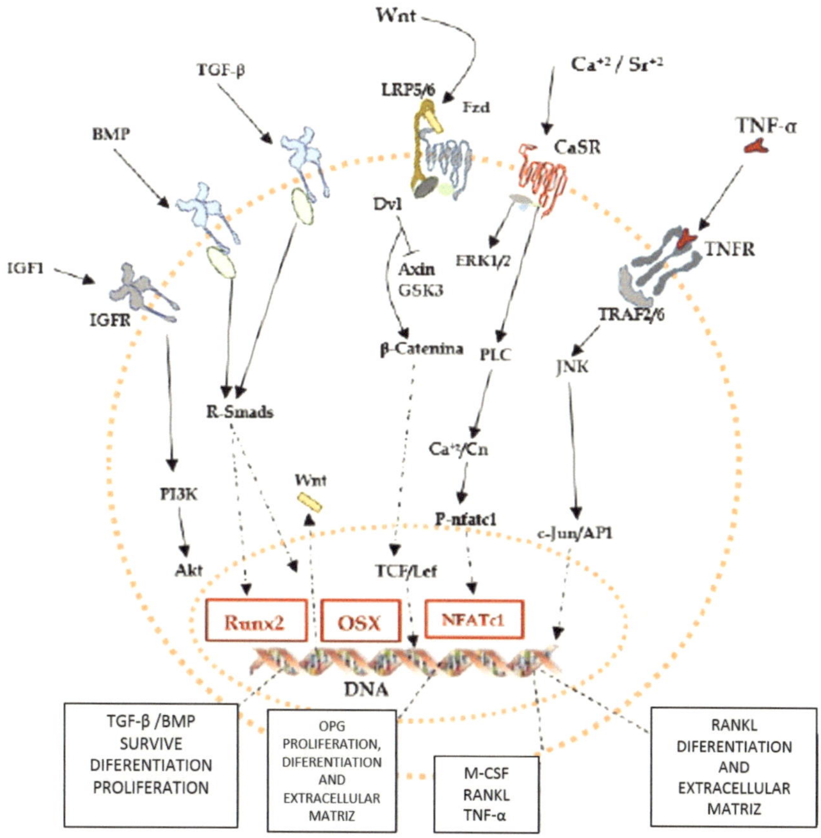

Figure 1.
Representative illustration of osteogenic signaling pathways. These pathways can activate several transcription factors, among them, RUNT (Runx 2), osterix (OSX), nuclear factor of activated T-cells 1 (NFATc1), and transcription factors of the Wnt pathway. Continuous arrows indicate interactions and signaling; dashed arrows indicate the actions described in boxes; and t-bar indicates block.

Manochantr et al. showed that after in vitro stimulation of bone marrow-derived MSCs with 100 ng/ml BMP-2, there was upregulation of the level of expression of genes associated with osteogenic differentiation (RUNX2 and OCN) and increase in alkaline phosphatase (ALP) production [46].

During a regular bone remodeling process, typical of an organism maintaining physiological stability, both BMPs and their antagonists are needed since BMPs induce osteo-precursor cells to proliferate and differentiate, thereby leading to formation of bone tissue. Members of the BMP family have different functions and are primarily related to the formation of bone and cartilage [47].

Upon BMP-receptor activation, receptor-regulated SMADs (R-SMADs) are translocated to the nucleus, where they regulate gene transcription by binding to DNA and interacting with DNA-binding proteins. Additionally, SMADs interact with transcription factors, transcriptional coactivators, and corepressors. The transcription factor associated with Runt-Runx is one of the most studied transcription factors for BMP signaling, responsible for regulating processes such as bone formation and hematopoiesis [46, 47].

Runx2 transcription factors cooperatively regulate gene transcription that lead to differentiation of mesenchymal progenitor cells into osteoblasts [48]. Hence, it is widely regarded as a marker for cells committed to the osteochondral lineage and osteoblast differentiation. Runx2 expression is low in mesenchymal cells and is induced by BMP signaling [49].

Osterix (OSX) is another example of a transcription factor mediated by BMP/SMAD signaling and likely by MAPK signaling and other pathways [50]. Taken together, Runx2 and Osterix are the most studied transcription factors for BMP signaling involved in the differentiation of MSCs into osteoblasts.

Moreover, recombinant BMP-2 (rhBMP-2) has been used for bone induction in humans being treated for long bone fractures and spinal arthrodesis [45]. A clinical study showed improved bone density and quantity formed when compared to the gold standard surgery (anterior iliac crest bone graft), used in maxilla reconstruction in cleft lip and palate patients.

3.2 Insulin-like growth factor type I

Insulin-like growth factor type I (IGF-1) is yet another factor currently being studied as an osteoinducer. IGF-1 is the most abundant growth factor found in the bone matrix and it plays an important role in development and maintenance of skeletal tissue [51]. It has been shown, under in vitro conditions, that IGF-1 is a stimulant for osteogenic differentiation through the increase in expression of ALP, Runx2, and OCN genes in MSCs from molar dental pulp [51].

Previous studies have demonstrated that the stimulant effect of IGF-1 on bone matrix synthesis in cell cultures derived from rat calvaria is a result of at least two distinct regulatory signals: first, the effect on cellular differentiation—osteoprogenitor cells and pre-osteoblasts—in osteoblasts (increased production of bone collagen); and second, the stimulation of osteoprogenitor cells' proliferation, thereby resulting in an increase in the number of functional osteoblasts. Despite working together to increase production of extracellular matrix, those signals differ in origin and can act synergistically with other factors, such as, for example, BMP-9 [37] and OSX, to promote osteogenic differentiation [50].

Insulin-like growth factors are known for mediating skeletal growth and bone formation [37, 52, 53]. Different studies have shown that IGF-1, in particular, promotes differentiation of bone cells in autocrine and paracrine pathways [52, 53]. Previous in vitro and in vivo studies have used IGF-1 to promote osteogenesis while treating dental pulp-derived osteoblastic cells [53, 54] and in an aged rat model, respectively. On the other hand, studies using rat fracture models show that the use of IGF-1 or PDGF alone does not stimulate OCN expression [55]. Nevertheless, using IGF-1 along with MSCs can cause expression of both factors to increase, as well as a significant upregulation of OCN by ODM in comparison to ODM alone.

The use of those factors for cell proliferation and differentiation is still being tested and is correlated with high treatment costs. On the other hand, low-level laser therapy (LLLT) could be a new alternative adjunct therapy for bone regeneration.

3.3 Low-level laser therapy

In the last 30 years, low-level laser therapy (LLLT) has been used mainly for the treatment of wounds; however, its applicability in pathological conditions such as tissue regeneration, pain relief, and inflammation has increased in different branches of regenerative medicine and dentistry [56, 57].

LLLT consists of exposing cells or tissues to low-level red and infrared lasers at wavelengths of 600–1100 nm and energy output of 1–500 mW and is called "low-level" due to its use of low-density light when compared to other forms of laser therapy. This type of irradiation may be a continuous or pulsed wave comprised of a constant, low-density energy beam (0.04–50 J/cm^2). The laser is directed at the target tissue or a monolayer of cells, with power in milliwatts (mW) [36, 58].

LLLT transmits energy at low levels; hence, there is no heat or sound emission nor vibrations. There are no thermal reactions because there is no immediate increase in temperature in the tissue being irradiated by laser. Experiments after low-level laser have shown negligible, immediate heat increase in tissue (±1°C) [36, 59].

Studies with LLLT have proven effective in biostimulation, increasing the rate of cell proliferation, migration, and adhesion. Several different lasers with varying sources of light—including helium-neon (HeNe), ruby, and gallium-aluminum-arsenide (GaAIA)—have been used in a range of LLLT treatments and protocols [36, 60–63].

As mentioned above, LLLT can promote a range of biological processes, including cell proliferation [59, 64, 65] and differentiation [36, 66]. The effects of LLLT on cell proliferation have been studied in vitro in several types of cells, namely: fibroblasts, endothelium, keratinocytes, myoblasts, and mesenchymal stem cells, among others [36, 66–71]. Nevertheless, the molecular mechanism associated with the stimulatory effects remains unclear.

One possible theory is the ability of LLLT to influence photoreceptors in cells. This mechanism is called photobiology or biostimulation. It has been stated that biostimulation occurs through the electron transport chain in mitochondrial enzymes, inducing high levels of cell respiration by endogenous porphyrin or cytochrome c during tissue stress (lesioned) [62], which increases cell metabolism and function [66]. The response to LLLT's biostimulation effects is an increase in microcirculation, leading to higher ATP production and subsequent increase in DNA and RNA synthesis, thereby improving cellular oxygenation, nutrition, and regeneration [59, 65].

Similar to any drug treatment, LLLT has its own "active ingredient," that is, its irradiation parameters, such as wavelength, power, power density, and energy density. Regarding interaction of the laser with matter, the effects of LLLT have been described by Karu [72] as: primary, acting as modulators of cell function, and secondary, relieving pain or inducing healing. Indeed, those effects depend on appropriate irradiation parameters [72].

Several mechanisms that aim at explaining the mitogenic effects of low-level laser therapy have been proposed, including: light absorption by mitochondrial enzymes; photon absorption by flavins and cytochromes in the mitochondrial respiratory chain, affecting electron transfer; singlet oxygen production through photoexcitation of endogenous porphyrins; and photoactivation of calcium channels, resulting in higher intracellular calcium concentrations and cell proliferation [73, 74].

Furthermore, laser therapy alters cell membrane permeability, causing subsequent physiological changes in the target cells. The magnitude of the biostimulation effect will depend on the wavelength used as well as the physiology of cell at the time [69].

It has been suggested that porphyrins and cytochromes, which are part of the mitochondrial respiratory chain, are the first photoreceptors in the visible wavelength range. When energy (photons) is absorbed by the photoreceptors' cell membrane, a cascade of cellular response occurs, provoking production of reactive oxygen species (ROS), ATP synthesis, changes in cell membrane permeability, and release of nitric oxide. Those effects in turn lead to an increase in cell proliferation; changes in extracellular matrix synthesis; and local effects in components of the immune, vascular, and nervous system. Besides, intracellular pH levels are altered—a change associated with activation of ATPase. Changes in oxidation-reduction status cause higher levels of intracellular Ca2 and stimulate cell metabolism. High levels of intracellular Ca2 promote several biological processes, such as RNA and DNA synthesis, cell mitosis, and secretion of proteins. It has been observed that Ca uptake by mammal cells can be induced by monochromatic red light (laser), depending on the dosage applied. Most cellular responses to LLLT derive from changes in mitochondrial and membrane activity, including mitochondrial membrane potential, as shown in **Figure 2**. Despite the positive results that argue for this type of treatment, the underlying action mechanism is yet to be understood [75].

In addition, studies show that ATP can activate P13K signaling pathway (phosphoinositide 3-kinase) through the ERK1/ERK2 genes, a pathway that regulates proliferation of certain types of cells [76]. Studies have also shown that LLLT promotes wound healing, collagen synthesis, nerve regeneration, bone remodeling and repair, and pain relief [57, 59, 77–80].

There are several studies in the literature that state the relationship between osteogenic differentiation, mesenchymal stem cells and LLLT, showing stimulation of matrix production, DNA synthesis, and formation of bone nodules in cultures of osteoblast-lineage cells after LLLT [36, 81, 82]. In 2005, Abramovitch-Gottlieb and colleagues used bone marrow MSCs cultured in 3D coralline (*Porites lutea*) biomaterial and He-Ne red laser irradiation (wavelength of 632.8 nm) to promote osteogenic differentiation [66]. Samples of biomaterial containing irradiated bone marrow MSCs showed an increase in neoformed bone tissue when compared to

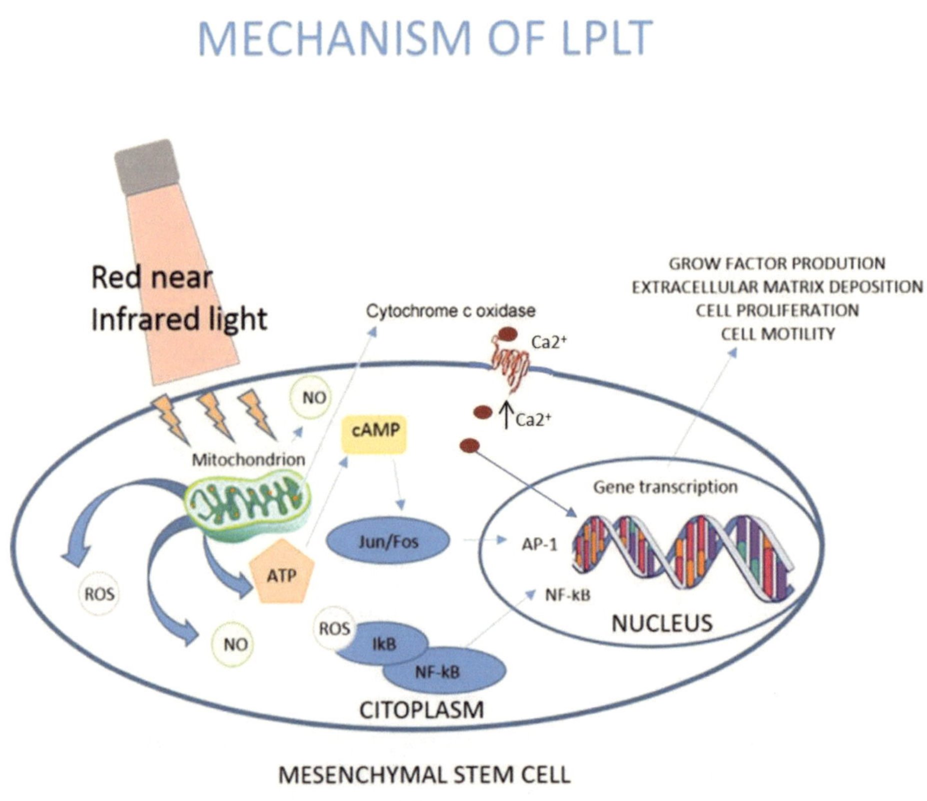

Figure 2.
The cellular effect of low-level laser therapy (LLLT) on cellular metabolism. LLLT is proposed to act via mitochondria (cytochrome c oxidase) displacing nitric oxide (NO) from the respiratory chain and increasing levels of adenosine triphosphate (ATP) and reactive oxygen species (ROS). These changes act via intermediaries cyclic adenosine monophosphate (cAMP)-activated transcription factors AP-1. The interaction of the ROS and IkB further transcription factor NF-κB. The LLLT can be photoactive of calcium channels, resulting in higher intracellular calcium concentrations. All stimuli resulting in changes in gene expression and subsequent downstream production of chemical messengers implicated in the cellular changes increase cell proliferation, cell differentiation, cell motility, and growth factors production.

non-irradiated samples. This suggests that tissue bioengineering (biomaterial containing mesenchymal stem cell) together with LLLT have biostimulation effects on osteogenic induction.

Osteogenic differentiation in MSCs has also been reinforced by another study using red laser at 647 nm. MSCs were irradiated with LLLT at differing periods of time and energy levels. Non-irradiated cells (control) were kept under the same conditions as irradiated cells. Samples of cells receiving LLLT showed a significant increase in production of extracellular matrix after 4–5 days compared to non-irradiated cells, indicating that red laser promotes osteoblast differentiation. This increase in extracellular production was maintained with daily irradiation (5, 10, and 20 J) for 21 days, which corresponds to the period of differentiation and maturation of MSCs in osteoblasts [36].

Moreover, in a study using a blue laser, MSCs were irradiated (wavelength of 405 nm) for 180 s through a fiber connected to the bottom of the culture plate. The results showed that irradiation with blue laser can promote extracellular calcification produced by MSCs differentiated into osteoblasts, in addition to inducing translocation of CRY1 protein (cryptochrome 1) from the cytoplasm to the nucleus. CRY1 is a regulator for circadian rhythm and extracellular calcification in MSCs [70]. Based on hypotheses described in previous studies, LLLT can act as adjunct treatment in tissue bioengineering, representing a new strategy in bone rehabilitation.

4. Final considerations

The creation of biobanks of mesenchymal stem cells due to the possibility of isolating and manipulating MSCs from a range of tissues as well as storing them in ultralow temperatures for future use as a bioengineering strategy for bone or other tissues' rehabilitation is of great economic and scientific interest. Yet, strategies and quality management of these biocomponents must still be developed.

The ability of MSCs for osteogenic differentiation has been well established in the literature; however, the analysis of the potential for differentiation between in vitro and in vivo sources of MSCs may direct their use in future therapies.

Author details

Carla Cristina Gomes Pinheiro and Daniela Franco Bueno*
Instituto de Ensino e Pesquisa do Hospital Sírio-Libanês, São Paulo, Brazil

*Address all correspondence to: dbuenousp@gmail.com

References

[1] Salmasi S, Nayyer L, Seifalian AM, Blunn GW. Nanohydroxyapatite effect on the degradation, osteoconduction and mechanical properties of polymeric bone tissue engineered scaffolds. The Open Orthopaedics Journal [Internet]. 2016;**10**:900-919. Available from: http://www.ncbi.nlm.nih.gov/pubmed/28217213 [Cited: September 24, 2018]

[2] Langer R, Vacanti J. Tissue engineering. Science. 1993 May 14;**260**(5110):920-926. Review. PubMed PMID: 8493529

[3] Gimbel M, Ashley RK, Sisodia M, Gabbay JS, Wasson KL, Heller J, et al. Repair of alveolar cleft defects: Reduced morbidity with bone marrow stem cells in a resorbable matrix. Journal of Craniofacial Surgery [Internet]. 2007;**18**(4):895-901. Available from: http://www.ncbi.nlm.nih.gov/pubmed/17667684 [Cited: November 6, 2016]

[4] Yousefi AM, James PF, Akbarzadeh R, Subramanian A, Flavin C, Oudadesse H. Prospect of stem cells in bone tissue engineering: A review. Stem Cells International [Internet]. 2016;**2016**:6180487. Available from: http://www.ncbi.nlm.nih.gov/pubmed/26880976 [Cited; November 6, 2016]

[5] Shanti RM, Li WJ, Nesti LJ, Wang X, Tuan RS. Adult mesenchymal stem cells: Biological properties, characteristics, and applications in maxillofacial surgery. Journal of Oral and Maxillofacial Surgery [Internet]. 2007;**65**(8):1640-1647. Available from: http://linkinghub.elsevier.com/retrieve/pii/S0278239107004715

[6] Raposo-Amaral CE, Bueno DF, Almeida AB, Jorgetti V, Costa CC, Gouveia CH, et al. Is bone transplantation the gold standard for repair of alveolar bone defects? Journal of Tissue Engineering [Internet]. 2014;**5**:2041731413519352. Available from: http://www.ncbi.nlm.nih.gov/pubmed/24551445%5Cnhttp://www.pubmedcentral.nih.gov/articlerender.fcgi?artid=PMC3924878

[7] Dimitriou R, Jones E, McGonagle D, Giannoudis PV. Bone regeneration: Current concepts and future directions. BMC Medicine [Internet]. 2011;**9**:66. Available from: http://www.ncbi.nlm.nih.gov/pubmed/21627784 [Cited: November 6, 2016]

[8] de Mendonca CA, Bueno DF, Martins MT, Kerkis I, Kerkis A, Fanganiello RD, et al. Reconstruction of large cranial defects in nonimmunosuppressed experimental design with human dental pulp stem cells. The Journal of Craniofacial Surgery. 2008;**19**(1):204-210

[9] Collas P, Cibelli JB, Stice SL, Golueke PJ, Munsie MJ, et al. Dedifferentiation of cells: New approaches. Cytotherapy. 1998;**9**(3):236-244

[10] Friedenstein AJ, Deriglasova UF, Kulagina NN, Panasuk AF, Rudakowa SF, Luriá EA, et al. Precursors for fibroblasts in different populations of hematopoietic cells as detected by the in vitro colony assay method. Experimental Hematology [Internet]. 1974;**2**(2):83-92. Available from: http://www.ncbi.nlm.nih.gov/pubmed/4455512 [Cited: November 6, 2016]

[11] Caplan AI. Mesenchymal stem cells. Journal of Orthopaedic Research [Internet]. 1991;**9**(5):641-650. Available from: http://doi.wiley.com/10.1002/jor.1100090504 [Cited: November 6, 2016]

[12] Friedenstein AJ, Gorskaja JF, Kulagina NN. Fibroblast precursors

in normal and irradiated mouse hematopoietic organs. Experimental Hematology [Internet]. 1976;**4**(5): 267-274. Available from: http://www.ncbi.nlm.nih.gov/pubmed/976387 [Cited: November 6, 2016]

[13] Zuk PA, Zhu M, Ashjian P, De Ugarte DA, Huang JI, Mizuno H, et al. Human adipose tissue is a source of multipotent stem cells. Molecular Biology of the Cell. 2002;**13**:4279-4295

[14] da Silva Meirelles L, Chagastelles PC. Mesenchymal stem cells reside in virtually all post-natal organs and tissues. Journal of Cell Science. 2006 Jun 1;**119**(Pt 11):2204-2213. [Epub 2006 May 9]. PubMed PMID: 16684817

[15] Jazedje T, Perin PM, Czeresnia CE, Maluf M, Halpern S, Secco M, et al. Human fallopian tube: A new source of multipotent adult mesenchymal stem cells discarded in surgical procedures. Journal of Translational Medicine [Internet]. 2009;**7**:46. Available from: http://www.pubmedcentral.nih.gov/articlerender.fcgi?artid=2714040&tool=pmcentrez&rendertype=abstract

[16] Bueno DF, Kerkis I, Costa AM, Martins MT, Kobayashi GS, Zucconi E, et al. New source of muscle-derived stem cells with potential for alveolar bone reconstruction in cleft lip and/or palate patients. Tissue Engineering Part A [Internet]. 2009;**15**(2): 427-435. Available from: http://www.liebertonline.com/doi/abs/10.1089/ten.tea.2007.0417 [Cited: November 9, 2016]

[17] Zucconi E, Vieira NM, Bueno CR Jr, Secco M, Jazedje T, Costa Valadares M, et al. Preclinical studies with umbilical cord mesenchymal stromal cells in different animal models for muscular dystrophy. Journal of Biomedicine and Biotechnology [Internet]. 2011;**2011**:715251. Available from: http://www.ncbi.nlm.nih.gov/entrez/query.fcgi?cmd=Retrieve&db=PubMed&dopt=Citation&list_uids=21785565

[18] Shi S, Bartold P, Miura M, Seo B, Robey P, Gronthos S. The efficacy of mesenchymal stem cells to regenerate and repair dental structures. Orthodontics & Craniofacial Research [Internet]. 2005;**8**(3):191-199. Available from: http://doi.wiley.com/10.1111/j.1601-6343.2005.00331.x [Cited: November 6, 2016]

[19] Dominici M, Le Blanc K, Mueller I, Slaper-Cortenbach I, Marini F, Krause D, et al. Minimal criteria for defining multipotent mesenchymal stromal cells. The International Society for Cellular Therapy Position Statement. Cytotherapy [Internet]. 2006;**8**(4): 315-317. Available from: http://www.ncbi.nlm.nih.gov/pubmed/16923606

[20] Kolf CM, Cho E, Tuan RS. Mesenchymal stromal cells. Biology of adult mesenchymal stem cells: Regulation of niche, self-renewal and differentiation. Arthritis Research & Therapy. 2007;**9**(1):204

[21] Kerkis I, Caplan AI. Stem cells in dental pulp of deciduous teeth. Tissue Engineering, Part B. Reviews [Internet]. 2012;**18**(2):129-138. Available from: http://www.ncbi.nlm.nih.gov/pubmed/22032258 [Cited: November 6, 2016]

[22] Secco M, Zucconi E, Vieira NM, Fogaça LLQ, Cerqueira A, Carvalho MDF, et al. Mesenchymal stem cells from umbilical cord: Do not discard the cord! Neuromuscular Disorders. 2008;**18**(1):17-18

[23] Kerkis I, Kerkis A, Dozortsev D, Stukart-Parsons GC, Gomes Massironi SM, Pereira LV, et al. Isolation and characterization of a population of immature dental pulp stem cells expressing OCT-4 and other embryonic stem cell markers. Cells Tissues Organs [Internet]. 2006;**184**(3-4):105-116. Available from: http://www.karger.com/doi/10.1159/000099617 [Cited: November 6, 2016]

[24] Collart-Dutilleul PY, Chaubron F, De Vos J, Cuisinier FJ. Allogenic banking of dental pulp stem cells for innovative therapeutics. World Journal of Stem Cells [Internet]. 2015;**7**(7):1010-1021. Available from: http://www.ncbi.nlm.nih.gov/pubmed/26328017 [Cited: November 6, 2016]

[25] Fernandes TL, Shimomura K, Asperti A, Pinheiro CCG, Caetano HVA, Oliveira CRGCM, et al. Development of a novel large animal model to evaluate human dental pulp stem cells for articular cartilage treatment. Stem Cell Reviews 2018 Oct;**14**(5):734-743. DOI: 10.1007/s12015-018-9820-2. PubMed PMID: 29728886; PubMed Central PMCID: PMC6132738

[26] Pittenger MF, Mackay AM, Beck SC, Jaiswal RK, Douglas R, Mosca JD, et al. Multilineage potential of adult human mesenchymal stem cells. Science [Internet]. 1999;**284**(5411):143-147. Available from: http://www.ncbi.nlm.nih.gov/pubmed/10102814 [Cited: November 6, 2016]

[27] Leyendecker A, CCG P, Amano MT, Bueno DF. The use of human mesenchymal stem cells as therapeutic agents for the in vivo treatment of immune-related diseases: A systematic review. Frontiers in Immunology. 2018;**9**(SEP):1-50

[28] Hibi H, Yamada Y, Ueda M, Endo Y. Alveolar cleft osteoplasty using tissue-engineered osteogenic material. International Journal of Oral and Maxillofacial Surgery. 2006;**35**(6):551-555

[29] Fanganiello RD, FAA I, Kobayashi GS, Alvizi L, Sunaga DY, Passos-Bueno MR. Increased in vitro osteopotential in SHED associated with higher IGF2 expression when compared with hASCs. Stem Cell Reviews and Reports [Internet]. 2015;**11**(4):635-644. Available from: http://link.springer.com/10.1007/s12015-015-9592-x [Cited: July 5, 2018]

[30] Gronthos S, Mankani M, Brahim J, Robey PG, Shi S. Postnatal human dental pulp stem cells (DPSCs) in vitro and in vivo. Proceedings of the National Academy of Sciences of the United States of America [Internet]. 2000;**97**(25):13625-13630. Available from: http://www.pnas.org/cgi/doi/10.1073/pnas.240309797 [Cited: August 30, 2018]

[31] Miura M, Gronthos S, Zhao M, Lu B, Fisher LW, Robey PG, et al. SHED:Stem cells from human exfoliated deciduous teeth. Proceedings of the National Academy of Sciences of the United States of America [Internet]. 2003;**100**(10):5807-5812. Available from: http://www.pubmedcentral.nih.gov/articlerender.fcgi?artid=156282&tool=pmcentrez&rendertype=abstract

[32] Leyendecker A Junior, Gomes Pinheiro CC, Lazzaretti Fernandes T, Franco Bueno D. The use of human dental pulp stem cells for in vivo bone tissue engineering: A systematic review. Journal of Tissue Engineering [Internet]. 2018;**9**:2041731417752766. Available from: http://www.ncbi.nlm.nih.gov/pubmed/29375756 [Cited: September 24, 2018]

[33] Fanganiello RD, Ishiy FAA, Kobayashi GS, Alvizi L, Sunaga DY, Passos-Bueno MR. Increased in vitro osteopotential in SHED associated with higher IGF2 expression when compared with hASCs. Stem Cell Reviews and Reports. 2015;**11**(4):635-644

[34] Moore ER, Zhu YX, Ryu HS, Jacobs CR. Periosteal progenitors contribute to load-induced bone formation in adult mice and require primary cilia to sense mechanical stimulation. Stem Cell Research & Therapy. 2018 Jul 11;**9**(1):190. DOI: 10.1186/s13287-018-0930-1. Erratum in: Stem Cell Res Ther. 2018 Aug 28;**9**(1):229. PubMed PMID: 29996901; PubMed Central PMCID: PMC6042447

[35] Debnath S, Yallowitz AR, McCormick J, Lalani S, Zhang T, Xu R, et al. Discovery of a periosteal stem cell mediating intramembranous bone formation. Nature [Internet]. 2018;**562**(7725):133-139. Available from: http://www.nature.com/articles/s41586-018-0554-8

[36] Pinheiro CCG, de Pinho MC, Aranha AC, Fregnani E, Bueno DF. Low power laser therapy: A strategy to promote the osteogenic differentiation of deciduous dental pulp stem cells from cleft lip and palate patients. Tissue Engineering Part A [Internet]. 2018;**24**(7-8):569-575. Available from: http://www.ncbi.nlm.nih.gov/pubmed/28699387 [Cited: August 13, 2018]

[37] Chen L, Zou X, Zhang RX, Pi CJ, Wu N, Yin LJ, et al. IGF1 potentiates BMP9-induced osteogenic differentiation in mesenchymal stem cells through the enhancement of BMP/Smad signaling. BMB Reports. 2016;**49**(2):122-127

[38] Alonso N, Risso GH, Denadai R, Raposo-Amaral CE. Effect of maxillary alveolar reconstruction on nasal symmetry of cleft lip and palate patients: A study comparing iliac crest bone graft and recombinant human bone morphogenetic protein-2. Journal of Plastic, Reconstructive & Aesthetic Surgery. 2014 Sep;**67**(9):1201-1208. DOI: 10.1016/j.bjps.2014.05.014. Epub 2014 May 20. PubMed PMID: 24909628

[39] Gao C, Peng S, Feng P, Shuai C. Bone biomaterials and interactions with stem cells. Bone research. 2017 Dec 21;**5**:17059. DOI: 10.1038/boneres.2017.59. eCollection 2017. Review. PubMed PMID: 29285402; PubMed Central PMCID: PMC5738879. Available from: www.nature. com/boneres [Cited: October 29, 2018]

[40] Paino F, La Noce M, Giuliani A, De Rosa A, Mazzoni S, Laino L, et al. Human DPSCs fabricate vascularized woven bone tissue: A new tool in bone tissue engineering. Clinical Science [Internet]. 2017;**131**:699-713. Available from: https://www.ncbi.nlm.nih.gov/pmc/articles/PMC5383003/pdf/cs1310699.pdf [Cited: October 19, 2018]

[41] Bessa PC, Casal M, Reis RL. Bone morphogenetic proteins in tissue engineering: the road from the laboratory to the clinic, part I (basic concepts). Journal of Tissue Engineering and Regenerative Medicine [Internet]. 2008;**2**(1):1-13. Available from: http://www.ncbi.nlm.nih.gov/pubmed/18293427 [Cited: August 30, 2018]

[42] Viti F, Landini M, Mezzelani A, Petecchia L, Milanesi L, Scaglione S. Osteogenic differentiation of MSC through calcium signaling activation: Transcriptomics and functional analysis. PLoS One. 2016;**11**(2):1-21

[43] Cho YD, Yoon WJ, Kim WJ, Woo KM, Baek JH, Lee G, et al. Epigenetic modifications and canonical wingless/int-1 class (WNT) signaling enable trans-differentiation of nonosteogenic cells into osteoblasts. The Journal of Biological Chemistry. 2014;**289**(29):20120-20128

[44] Chen Q, Liu W, Sinha KM, Yasuda H, de Crombrugghe B. Identification and characterization of microRNAs controlled by the osteoblast-specific transcription factor osterix. PLoS One. 2013;**8**(3):e58104. DOI: 10.1371/journal.pone.0058104. [Epub 2013 Mar 5]. PubMed PMID: 23472141; PubMed Central PMCID: PMC3589352

[45] Canan LW, da Silva FR, Alonso N, Tanikawa DYS, Rocha DL, Coelho JCU. Human bone morphogenetic protein-2 use for maxillary reconstruction in cleft lip and palate patients. Journal of Craniofacial Surgery [Internet]. 2012;**23**(6):1627-1633. Available from: http://www.ncbi.nlm.nih.gov/pubmed/23147291

[46] Manochantr S, Marupanthorn K, Tantrawatpan C, Kheolamai P, Tantikanlayaporn D, Sanguanjit P. The effects of BMP-2, miR-31, miR-106a, and miR-148a on osteogenic differentiation of MSCs derived from amnion in comparison with MSCs derived from the bone marrow. Stem Cells International. 2017;**2017**

[47] James AW. Review of signaling pathways governing MSC osteogenic and adipogenic differentiation. Scientifica (Cairo) [Internet]. 2013;**2013**:684736. Available from: http://www.pubmedcentral.nih.gov/articlerender.fcgi?artid=3874981&tool=pmcentrez&rendertype=abstract

[48] Zhang Y-W, Yasui N, Ito K, Huang G, Fujii M, Hanai J-I, et al. A RUNX2/PEBP2αA/CBFA1 mutation displaying impaired transactivation and Smad interaction in cleidocranial dysplasia. Proceedings of the National Academy of Sciences of the USA. 2000 Sep 12;**97**(19):10549-10554. Published online: 2000 Aug 29. DOI: 10.1073/pnas.180309597. PMCID: PMC27062

[49] Maeda S, Hayashi M, Komiya S, Imamura T, Miyazono K. Endogenous TGF-b signaling suppresses maturation of osteoblastic mesenchymal cells. The EMBO Journal [Internet]. 2004;**23**:552-563. Available from: www.embojournal.org [Cited: August 13, 2018]

[50] Celil AB, Hollinger JO, Campbell PG. Osx transcriptional regulation is mediated by additional pathways to BMP2/Smad signaling. Journal of Cellular Biochemistry [Internet]. 2005;**95**(3):518-528. Available from: http://doi.wiley.com/10.1002/jcb.20429 [Cited: August 13, 2018]

[51] Alkharobi H, Alhodhodi A, Hawsawi Y, Alkafaji H, Devine D, El-Gendy R, et al. IGFBP-2 and -3 co-ordinately regulate IGF1 induced matrix mineralisation of differentiating human dental pulp cells. Stem Cell Research. Nov 2016;**17**(3):517-522. DOI: 10.1016/j.scr.2016.09.026

[52] Wang S, Mu J, Fan Z, Yu Y, Yan M, Lei G, et al. Insulin-like growth factor 1 can promote the osteogenic differentiation and osteogenesis of stem cells from apical papilla. Stem Cell Research [Internet]. 2012;**8**(3):346-356. Available from: http://dx.doi.org/10.1016/j.scr.2011.12.005

[53] Feng X, Huang D, Lu X, Feng G, Xing J, Lu J, et al. Insulin-like growth factor 1 can promote proliferation and osteogenic differentiation of human dental pulp stem cells via mTOR pathway. Development, Growth & Differentiation [Internet]. 2014;**56**(9):615-624. Available from: http://doi.wiley.com/10.1111/dgd.12179

[54] Siddals KW, Allen J, Sinha S, Canfield AE, Kalra PA, Martin Gibson J. Apposite insulin-like growth factor (IGF) receptor glycosylation is critical to the maintenance of vascular smooth muscle phenotype in the presence of factors promoting osteogenic differentiation and mineralization. The Journal of Biological Chemistry. 2011;**286**(19):16623-16630

[55] Commons GW, Longaker MT. Regulation of human adipose-derived stromal cell osteogenic differentiation by insulin-like growth factor-1 and platelet- derived growth factor-alpha. 2011;**126**(1):41-52

[56] Conlan MJ, Rapley JW, Cobb CW. Biostimulation of wound healing by low-energy laser irradiation. Journal of Clinical Periodontology [Internet]. 1996;**23**:492-196. ISSN: 0303-6979. Available from: https://onlinelibrary.wiley.com/doi/pdf/10.1111/j.1600-051X.1996.tb00580.x [Cited: July 23, 2018]

[57] Nanami T, Shiba H, Ikeuchi S, Nagai T, Asanami S, Shibata T. Clinical applications and basic studies of laser in dentistry and

oral surgery. The Keio Journal of Medicine [Internet]. 1993;**42**(4):199-201. Available from: http://www.ncbi.nlm.nih.gov/pubmed/8126980 [Cited: November 6, 2016]

[58] Stein A, Benayahu D, Maltz L, Oron U. Low-level laser irradiation promotes proliferation and differentiation of human osteoblasts in vitro. Photomedicine and Laser Surgery [Internet]. 2005;**23**(2):161-166. Available from: http://www.ncbi.nlm.nih.gov/pubmed/15910179 [Cited: November 6, 2016]

[59] Conlan MJ, Rapley JW, Cobb CM. Biostimulation of wound healing by low-energy laser irradiation. A review. Journal of Clinical Periodontology [Internet]. 1996;**23**(5):492-496. Available from: http://www.ncbi.nlm.nih.gov/pubmed/8783057 [Cited: November 6, 2016]

[60] Tajali SB, Macdermid JC, Houghton P, Grewal R. Effects of low power laser irradiation on bone healing in animals: A meta-analysis. Journal of Orthopaedic Surgery and Research. 4 Jan 2010;**5**:1. DOI: 10.1186/1749-799X-5-1. PubMed PMID: 20047683; PubMed Central PMCID: PMC2829511

[61] Fekrazad R, Sadeghi Ghuchani M, Eslaminejad M, Taghiyar L, Kalhori KA, Pedram M, et al. The effects of combined low level laser therapy and mesenchymal stem cells on bone regeneration in rabbit calvarial defects. Journal of Photochemistry and Photobiology B: Biology. 2015 Oct;**151**:180-185. DOI: 10.1016/j.jphotobiol.2015.08.002. [Epub 2015 Aug 11]. PubMed PMID: 26298068

[62] Karu T, Pyatibrat L, Kalendo G. Irradiation with He Ne laser increases ATP level in cells cultivated in vitro. Journal of Photochemistry and Photobiology B: Biology. 1995;**27**(3):219-223

[63] Yu H-S, Chang K-L, Yu C-L, Chen J-W, Chen G-S. Low-energy helium-neon laser irradiation stimulates interleukin-la and interleukin-8 release from cultured human keratinocytes. Journal of Investigative Dermatology. 1996 Oct;**107**(4):593-596. PubMed PMID: 8823366

[64] Stein E, Koehn J, Sutter W, Wendtlandt G, Wanschitz F, Thurnher D, et al. Initial effects of low-level laser therapy on growth and differentiation of human osteoblast-like cells. Wiener Klinische Wochenschrift. 2008;**120**(3-4):112-117

[65] AlGhamdi KM, Kumar A, Moussa NA. Low-level laser therapy: A useful technique for enhancing the proliferation of various cultured cells. Lasers in Medical Science [Internet]. 2012;**27**(1):237-249. Available from: http://link.springer.com/10.1007/s10103-011-0885-2 [Cited: November 6, 2016]

[66] Abramovitch-Gottlib L, Gross T, Naveh D, Geresh S, Rosenwaks S, Bar I, et al. Low level laser irradiation stimulates osteogenic phenotype of mesenchymal stem cells seeded on a three-dimensional biomatrix. Lasers in Medical Science [Internet]. 2005;**20**(3-4):138-146. Available from: http://link.springer.com/10.1007/s10103-005-0355-9 [Cited: November 9, 2016]

[67] Hrnjak M, Kuljić-Kapulica N, Budisin A, Giser A. Stimulatory effect of low-power density He-Ne laser radiation on human fibroblasts in vitro. Vojnosanitetski Pregled [Internet];**52**(6):539-546. Available from: http://www.ncbi.nlm.nih.gov/pubmed/8644477 [Cited: November 6, 2016]

[68] Góralczyk K, Szymańska J, Łukowicz M, Drela E, Kotzbach R, Dubiel M, et al. Effect of LLLT on endothelial cells culture. Lasers in Medical Science. 2014;**30**(1):273-278

[69] Yu HS, Chang KL, Yu CL, Chen JW, Chen GS. Low-energy helium-neon laser irradiation stimulates interleukin-1 alpha and interleukin-8 release from cultured human keratinocytes. Journal of Investigative Dermatology [Internet]. 1996;**107**(4):593-596. PubMed PMID: 8823366. Available from: http://www.ncbi.nlm.nih.gov/pubmed/8823366 [Cited: November 6, 2016]

[70] Kushibiki T, Awazu K. Blue laser irradiation enhances extracellular calcification of primary mesenchymal stem cells. Photomedicine and Laser Surgery [Internet]. 2009;**27**(3):493-498. Available from: http://www.liebertonline.com/doi/abs/10.1089/pho.2008.2343 [Cited: November 6, 2016]

[71] Kushibiki T, Hirasawa T, Okawa S, Ishihara M. Low reactive level laser therapy for mesenchymal stromal cells therapies. Stem Cells International. 2015;**2015**

[72] Karu T. Primary and secondary mechanisms of action of visible to near-IR radiation on cells. Journal of Photochemistry and Photobiology B: Biology [Internet]. 1999;**49**(1): 1-17. Available from: https://www.sciencedirect.com/science/article/pii/S101113449800219X?via%3Dihub [Cited: September 24, 2018]

[73] Nagata MJH, Santinoni CS, Pola NM, de Campos N, Messora MR, Bomfim SRM, et al. Bone marrow aspirate combined with low-level laser therapy: A new therapeutic approach to enhance bone healing. Journal of Photochemistry and Photobiology B: Biology. 2013;**121**:6-14

[74] Marques MM, Diniz IMA, de Cara SPHM, Pedroni ACF, Abe GL, D'Almeida-Couto RS, et al. Photobiomodulation of dental derived mesenchymal stem cells: A systematic review. Photomedicine and Laser Surgery [Internet]. 2016;**34**(11): 500-508. Available from: http://online.liebertpub.com/doi/10.1089/pho.2015.4038

[75] Zungu IL, Hawkins Evans D, Abrahamse H. Mitochondrial responses of normal and injured human skin fibroblasts following low level laser irradiation—An in vitro study. Photochemistry and Photobiology [Internet]. 2009;**85**(4):987-996. Available from: http://doi.wiley.com/10.1111/j.1751-1097.2008.00523.x [Cited: September 24, 2018]

[76] Li C-S, Zheng Z, Su XX, Wang F, Ling M, Zou M. Activation of the extracellular signal-regulated kinase signaling is critical for human umbilical cord mesenchymal stem cell osteogenic differentiation. BioMed Research International. 2016;**2016**:3764372. DOI: 10.1155/2016/3764372. [Epub 2016 Feb 16]. PubMed PMID: 26989682; PubMed Central PMCID: PMC4771893

[77] Tim CR, Bossini PS, Kido HW, Malavazi I, von Zeska Kress MR, Carazzolle MF, et al. Effects of low-level laser therapy on the expression of osteogenic genes during the initial stages of bone healing in rats: A microarray analysis. Lasers in Medical Science. 2015;**30**(9):2325-2333

[78] Silva GBL, Sacono NT, Othon-Leite AF, Mendonça EF, Arantes AM, Bariani C, et al. Effect of low-level laser therapy on inflammatory mediator release during chemotherapy-induced oral mucositis: A randomized preliminary study. Lasers in Medical Science. 2014;**30**(1):117-126

[79] Anders JJ, Borke RC, Woolery SK, Van de Merwe WP. Low power laser irradiation alters the rate of regeneration of the rat facial nerve. Lasers in Surgery and Medicine [Internet]. 1993;**13**(1): 72-82. Available from: http://www.ncbi.nlm.nih.gov/pubmed/8426530 [Cited: November 6, 2016]

[80] Huang YY, Chen AC, Carroll JD, Hamblin MR. Biphasic dose response in low level light therapy. Dose Response. 1 Sep 2009;**7**(4):358-383. DOI: 10.2203/dose-response.09-027. Hamblin. PubMed PMID: 20011653; PubMed Central. PMCID: PMC2790317

[81] Tim CR, KNZ P, BRO R, Fernandes K, Matsumoto MA, Parizotto NA, et al. Low-level laser therapy enhances the expression of osteogenic factors during bone repair in rats. Lasers in Medical Science [Internet]. 2014;**29**(1):147-156. Available from: http://link.springer.com/10.1007/s10103-013-1302-9 [Cited: July 23, 2018]

[82] Pereira LO, JPF L, Azevedo RB, Gronthos S, Mankani M, Brahim J, et al. Laser irradiation did not increase the proliferation or the differentiation of stem cells from normal and inflamed dental pulp. Archives of Oral Biology [Internet]. 2012;**57**(8):1079-1085. Available from: http://www.ncbi.nlm.nih.gov/pubmed/22469390 [Cited: November 6, 2016]

Chapter 7

Distraction Osteogenesis in Oral and Craniomaxillofacial Reconstructive Surgery

Firdaus Hariri, Siok Yoong Chin, Jonathan Rengarajoo, Qi Chao Foo, Siti Nur Nabihah Zainul Abidin and Ahmad Fadhli Ahmad Badruddin

Abstract

Distraction osteogenesis (DO) is a tissue engineering method to regenerate new bone. The application of DO in the field of oral and craniomaxillofacial surgery has provided a promising alternative as it can be integrated with conventional surgical technique for bone lengthening or expansion. This technique has the advantages of providing superior amount of bone lengthening thus eliminating the need of autogenous graft and donor site morbidity, can be applied in young patients and allows simultaneous expansion of the surrounding soft tissues. In this chapter, we provide a comprehensive overview of the background history and development of DO which is based on Ilizarov technique, along with its basic principles, indications, classification of DO devices and protocol in craniomaxillofacial bone lengthening or expansion. Its clinical applications which include alveolar DO, mandible DO, maxilla DO, transport DO and craniofacial DO are clarified. This technique however requires proper understanding of clinical and technical components to avoid potential complications which include relapse, infection, adjacent structure injury, device failure and other complications. The emerging results of research and advances in DO are further elaborated at the end of this chapter.

Keywords: distraction osteogenesis, craniomaxillofacial, craniofacial surgery, bone lengthening, osteodistraction

1. Introduction

Distraction osteogenesis (DO) is a tissue engineering method and can be integrated with various craniomaxillofacial surgical techniques to generate new bone via stretching the surgically osteotomized bone with the aid of a mechanical device that is designed to control both the traction rate and the movement vector. This technique utilizes the fundamental healing properties of the human body by inducing regeneration and remodeling of callus between osteotomized site, also known as distraction gap. Callus between the distraction gap will be stretched with the aid of the distraction device to apply a uniform traction force thus allowing formation of new bone. Distraction osteogenesis does not only cause creation of new bone but also stimulates a process called neohistogenesis, where the surrounding soft tissue simultaneously expand and cover the newly formed callus.

The evolution of DO technique in clinical application which was first introduced in orthopedics field has now been widely applied as treatment alternative in cranio-maxillofacial region particularly for the management of congenital and acquired complex craniofacial structural defects. These complex structural defects involve conditions such as severely atrophic alveolar ridge, micrognathia (small mandible) or maxillary hypoplasia leading to respiratory issue as well as complex craniofacial deformities causing restriction of intracranial space and potential eye problems. The application of DO allows superior structural expansion and bone lengthening to restore the important functional discrepancies associated with these deformities.

2. History

Most novel approach in medical field evolved from the requirement of its clinical demand. Based on ancient records, Hippocrates was the first to come up with ideas of bone fracture reduction and stabilization. **Table 1** below summarizes the evolving history of DO.

In craniomaxillofacial region, the first clinical application of DO was reported by McCarthy in 1992 for mandibular lengthening. The success of mandibular lengthening has paved ways for many other craniomaxillofacial DO indications involving other regions such as the alveolar ridge, maxilla, and midface, as well as in cranial vault expansion.

3. Principles of distraction osteogenesis

3.1 Basic principles

In a normal fracture healing, soft callus formation (callotasis) allows the fracture site to heal. With this principle, DO involves the manipulation of this callus in the distraction chamber for structural lengthening before calcification occurs.

Corticotomy is a process where an osteotomy to the cortical layer of the bone is performed in order separate the segments while at the same time preserving the blood supply to the bone from the medulla and periosteum. Distraction rate in DO

Year	Surgeon	Advancement
1860	Dr. Angell [2]	Threaded jackscrew attached to both premolar transpalatally to obtain expansion over the maxillary suture
1905	Codivilla	Femoral bone extension using axial forces – serial application of casts that we pulled with the aid of the bed frame traction.
1927	Abbot	Replaced the multiple cast with pins inserted on the femur and used springs to aid in distraction
1948	Allan	Screw device was incorporated to control the rate of distraction (technique was abandoned due to multiple complications)
1950	Ilizarov [3, 4]	Corticotomy with minimal insult to the surrounding blood supply and using tension ring fixators to control distraction
1973	Snyder et al.	Mandibular lengthening in a canine animal model
1992	McCarthy et al.	First series of successful distraction in human mandible – the start of distraction osteogenesis technique for craniofacial deformities

Table 1.
The history and evolution of distraction osteogenesis [1].

describes the distance in millimeter (mm) in which the bone is moved per day and distraction rhythm describes the frequency of device activation per day.

Distraction osteogenesis comprises of three sequential phases; latency, distraction and consolidation phase which is distinct in every aspect. These phases are simplified in the illustration below (**Figure 1**).

a. Latency phase: A time period which is required for the formation of callus. Ilizarov suggested 5–7 days, but this depends on the microvasculature and physiological state of bone formation over the distraction site. At cellular level, there is hypoxia occurring over the osteotomized structure inducing angiogenic respond and migration of mesenchymal cells to help produce collagen synthesis. Latency period should be short enough to prevent calcification and long enough for adequate callus formation.

b. Distraction phase: To achieve target bone growth, the rigid distraction device needs to be activated as per suggested protocol. The device is activated via turning axial screw with a movement of 0.25–0.5 mm (depends on the system used) per turn. The success of the distraction depends on the rate and frequency of the distraction. If the distraction is carried out fast by increasing the rate and frequency it may lead to ischemia at the cellular level causing malunion over the distraction site. In contrary, reduced rate and frequency may lead to early ossification, thus indirectly causing complication to the distraction. Clinicians worldwide tend to keep the frequency to 2–4 times of activation daily with the target of 1.0–1.5 mm distraction rate per day. Histologically, 10–14 days post distraction, osteoid synthesis starts at the margin of the osteotomized bone adjacent to the blood vessels [5]. At around 3 weeks post distraction, progressive calcification starts to form bone spicules.

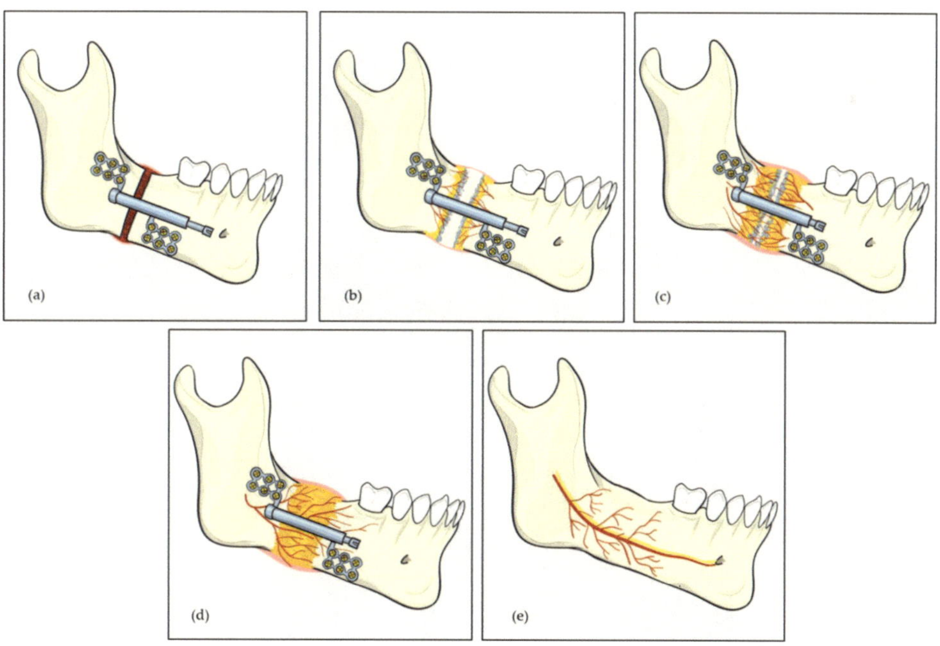

Figure 1.
The phases of distraction osteogenesis. (a) Latency period in which hematoma formation occurs following osteotomy which is later replaced by granulation tissue. (b) During distraction period, bone gap is progressively increased with osteogenesis at the margin of distraction gap. (c) Osteogenesis extend to the Centre of the gap during consolidation phase. (d) Maturation of the ossification in the distraction chamber in late consolidation period. (e) Bone remodeling and continuity of alveolar canal after completion of distraction osteogenesis.

c. Consolidation phase: This phase entails a long period of immobilization where the stretched callus is allowed to mature with the support of the device, keeping the callus in a stretched and stable position as well as preventing cartilaginous intermediate. Remodeling starts by allowing the formation of lamella bone with bone marrow elements over a period of time. The duration of the consolidation phase is around 4–12 weeks with 8 weeks being the average. Clinically, it is suggested that the consolidation phase is kept at twice as long as the activation phase and the timing of the consolidation period depends on the location of the distraction site and rate of bone metabolism [6].

Even though there is a variation of value for latency phase, rate and rhythms of distraction as well as duration of consolidation phase, most protocols are based on Ilizarov principle and in addition, tailored specifically according to the site of distraction, type of device used, surrounding soft tissue resistance and rate of bone metabolism. Meticulous planning using 3-dimensional surgical model (**Figure 2**) with a simulated activation will help gauge the required length of distraction as well as anticipating potential complications that may arise throughout the treatment.

3.2 Classification of distractor devices

Distractor devices are generally classified as external or internal. External device is bone-borne, consisting of fixation clamps and distraction rods which are attached to the bone by percutaneous pins. Internal device can be placed subcutaneously or intraorally, and subdivided into bone-borne, tooth-borne or hybrid (a combination of bone-borne and tooth-borne).

The devices are available in different vectors of distraction. Most commonly used is unidirectional or single vector distractor. There are also bidirectional, multidirectional

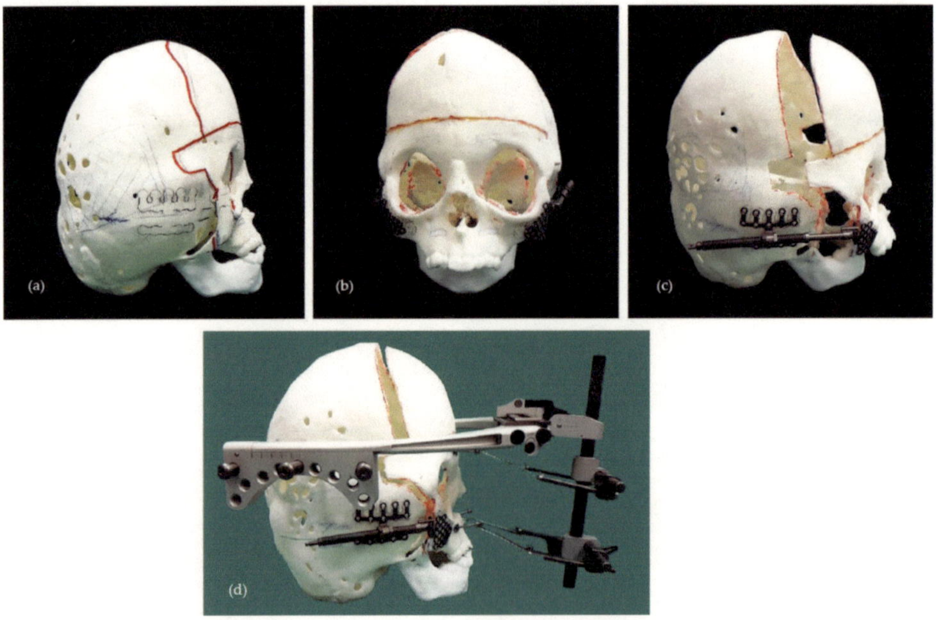

Figure 2.
Surgical simulation for DO procedure using stereolithography (STL) model for craniofacial distraction in AP direction. (a) Red line markings indicate the planned osteotomy line. (b) Placement of internal devices at zygoma area bilaterally, parallel in the horizontal plane. (c) Distraction simulation on STL model to confirm correct direction and final position of distracted midfacial bone. (d) Placement of external device to distribute the distraction forces equally to supraorbital and maxillary region, therefore increasing the distraction stability.

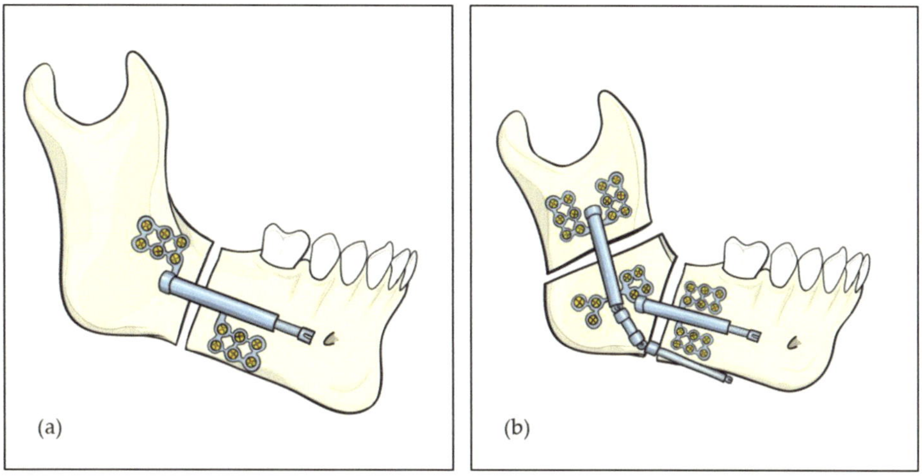

Figure 3.
Different designs for distractor devices according to its vector. (a) Unidirectional distractor (b) Bidirectional distractor.

and curvilinear distractors (**Figure 3**). External device allows better vector control in multidirectional lengthening with adjustment possible during the distraction period [7]. Internal devices carry less morbidity but both types of distractor device are associated with their own complications as described later in this chapter.

The choice of distractor depends on the site of device application, vector of distraction path, magnitude of movement, patient's factors such as age, medical comorbidities, financial as well as surgeon's preference. The advantages and disadvantages of external and internal distractor devices [8, 9] are described in **Table 2** below.

3.3 Indications

Generally, DO in craniomaxillofacial region is indicated for superior bone lengthening, expansion or augmentation in which, conventional methods may have limitations. The direction of augmentation or expansion may vary from vertical, anterior–posterior (AP), transverse or multi-directional.

In pediatric population, DO is used in syndromic craniosynostosis cases where there is a functional need to increase the size of intracranial volume and orbital cavities to relieve increased intracranial pressure (ICP) and severe exorbitism,

	Advantages	Disadvantages
External device	Multidirectional lengthening with angular adjustment possible during distraction	Patient apprehension to wear bulky external devices
	Relatively simple to apply intraoperatively	Potential permanent facial scarring
	Easy for patient to activate	
	Can be removed without the need for second operative procedure	
Internal device	Absence of facial scars	Design limitations due to limited size of device and restricted access to oral cavity
	Inconspicuous nature of device	
	Better stability of device to bone	

Table 2.
Advantages and disadvantages between external and internal distractor.

respectively. Obstructive sleep apnea (OSA) resulting from midfacial retrusion or hypoplastic mandible is another indication for DO in children.

In adult patients with severe mandibular or maxillary deficiency in which correction cannot be achieved via conventional orthognathic surgery, DO is recommended. It is also used for correction of hemifacial microsomia and in bone transport technique, for example to reconstruct a hypoplastic or resected mandibular condyle.

Distraction of atrophic alveolar ridges can be performed to increase the width or height of alveolar bone, hence creating adequate bone for dental implant insertion without the need for autogenous bone graft. These indications are summarized in **Table 3**.

3.4 Protocol

There is a wide variation in the protocol of craniomaxillofacial distraction. Following osteotomy, latency period ranges from 3 to 7 days [10]. Standard activation rate is 1 mm per day. Faster rate may cause incomplete osteogenesis or fibrous union while slower rate may result in premature ossification [11].

However, successful distraction in pediatric population has been reported with latency period as little as 24 hours [12, 13], owing to significant vascularity and healing potential in young bone. In addition, distraction of 2 mm per day is proven safe and provide similar success rate as 1 mm per day in children younger than 12 months [14].

Rhythm of activation can be adjusted based on manufacturer's design of activation rod. One full turn may represent 0.35, 0.5 or 1.0 mm. Therefore, amount of desired daily bone lengthening can be divided throughout the day instead of single activation to produce higher bone quality in terms of volume and architecture. Amid this, an experimental study by Djasim et al. [15] concluded that an increase in rhythm from one to three activations daily does not create significantly more bone. With the advent of automated device for continuous distraction, it allows bone fill at faster distraction rate compared to discontinuous distraction [16].

Site of DO	Direction of DO	Conditions
Mandible	Vertical (Ridge) Width (Ridge) Lengthening (Body) Vertical (Ramus) Transverse (Symphysis)	Severely atrophic ridge Knife edge ridge Micrognathia Hemifacial microsomia Micrognathia in transverse
Maxilla	Vertical (Ridge) Advancement Transverse	Severely atrophic ridge Maxillary hypoplasia in AP (craniofacial syndrome, cleft maxilla) Maxillary hypoplasia in transverse
Craniofacial	Posterior expansion Fronto-orbital Monobloc	Syndromic craniosynostosis (increased in ICP) Syndromic craniosynostosis (increased in ICP, severe exorbitism) Syndromic craniosynostosis (increased in ICP, severe exorbitism, OSA)
Other: Transport Reconstructed jaw	Vertical Anterior–posterior (AP) Vertical	Facial cleft Zygoma Severe alveolar ridge defect (trauma, post-ablative) Vascularized or non-vascularized reconstructed jaw (e.g. fibula, iliac, etc.)

Table 3.
Summary of indications for DO.

Period of consolidation is based upon the length of bony distraction. An experimental study on dog mandible by Smith et al. [17] demonstrated that minimum time for bone regenerate to mineralize is 6–8 weeks, however they suggested that this period should be extended up to 10 or 12 weeks in human population. The authors also discussed that the Ilizarov protocol which was based on long bone lengthening of allowing 2 days of consolidation for each millimeter of distraction does not apply in craniomaxillofacial bone. As craniomaxillofacial bone distraction is shorter in length as compared to lower limb distraction, it is less mineralized at the beginning of consolidation period therefore needing a longer consolidation period. Whereas in long bones, due to more length of distraction, mineralization of regenerate would have started during distraction period itself resulting in less regenerate needed to be mineralized during consolidation period itself.

Most commonly practiced consolidation period for craniomaxillofacial region is 12 weeks [18, 19]. This duration may be lengthened based on surgeon's clinical judgment such as in syndromic craniosynostosis cases. However, to accommodate patient's and parents' schedule, distraction devices are often removed well past the determined consolidation period.

4. Clinical application

4.1 Alveolar DO

In deficient alveolar bone height for implant placement, DO could increase bone level up to 16 mm at the rate of 1 mm per day (**Figure 4**). However, comprehensive assessment is required in a severely resorbed ridge as minimal thickness for both basal and transport segment are necessary for the fixation of the distractor plates. It is also very important to ensure the lingual or palatal mucosa remains intact to the transport segment for vascularization.

4.2 Mandibular DO

In micrognathia or mandibular hypoplasia in anterior–posterior (AP) direction, DO can be considered when superior mandibular body lengthening is needed

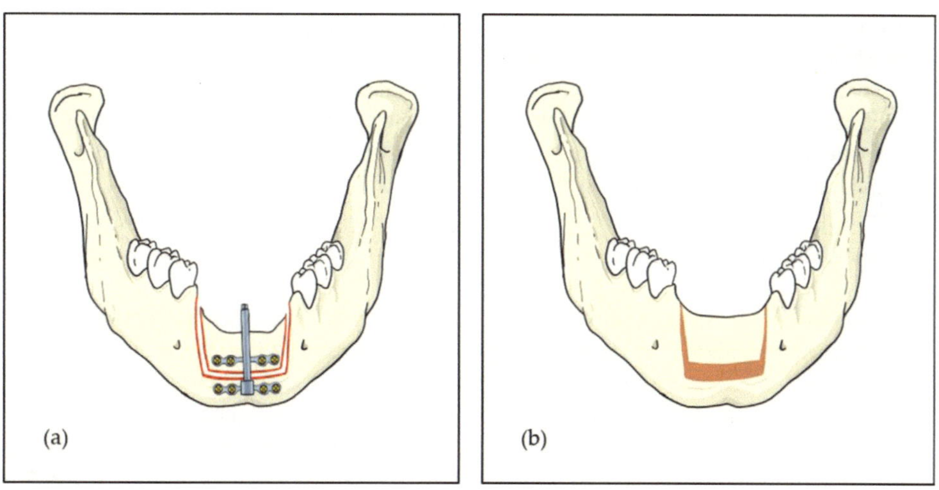

Figure 4.
Alveolar DO for atrophic mandibular anterior ridge. (a) Application of internal device for vertical distraction. (b) New height of distracted alveolar ridge.

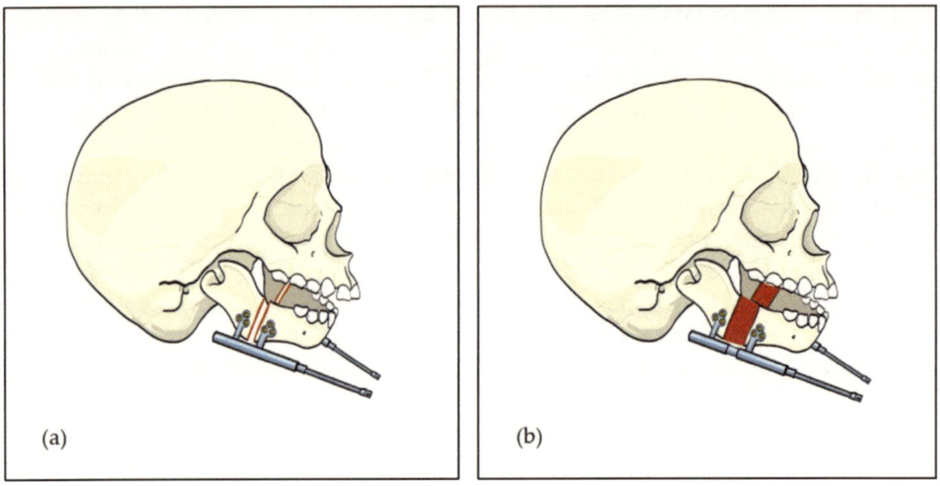

Figure 5.
Example of mandibular DO for hypoplastic mandible. (a) Application of internal distractor device in parallelism for bilateral mandibular lengthening. (b) Distracted mandible in AP direction.

(**Figure 5**). In comparison, a conventional bilateral sagittal split osteotomy may allow up to 10 mm of jaw lengthening while up to 30 mm advancement could be achieved with DO subjected to the size of device [20].

Mandibular DO is often indicated in cases of OSA secondary to conditions such as Treacher Collins syndrome and non-syndromic micrognathia. Improvement in apnea hypopnea index (AHI) score could be seen after 15 mm of DO and the distraction could continue up to 25 mm until an acceptable AHI of less than 5 is achieved [20]. However, the determination of distraction vector is paramount as deviated mandibular arch position at the end of distraction procedure may lead to severe malocclusion. Precaution is also needed intra-operatively as the osteotomy carries the risk of inferior dental nerve injury.

4.3 Maxillary DO

This technique can be applied for maxillary advancement in patients with OSA secondary to severe maxillary or midface hypoplasia (**Figure 6**). Other condition such as cleft maxillary hypoplasia may also need superior segmental advancement to correct the class III jaw discrepancy. Traditional Le Fort I osteotomy with superior advancement may carry the risk of significant relapse due to scar formation and soft tissue memory [21]. DO allows controlled soft tissue expansion and consolidation period thus reducing this problem.

4.4 Transport DO

Transport DO can be indicated in a condition where significant defect is presence (**Figure 7**). Defect can be secondary to post-ablative procedure such as in maxillectomy, huge cyst enucleation or congenital condition such as in facial cleft. Comprehensive planning is important as the pre-determination of osteotomy design and vector is paramount in ensuring the right position for the transported segment is achieved at the targeted opposing bony region. The challenging aspect of transport DO is to ensure the vascularity and maintaining an intact distraction chamber as failure to do so may lead to transport segment resorption resulting to a more severe defect.

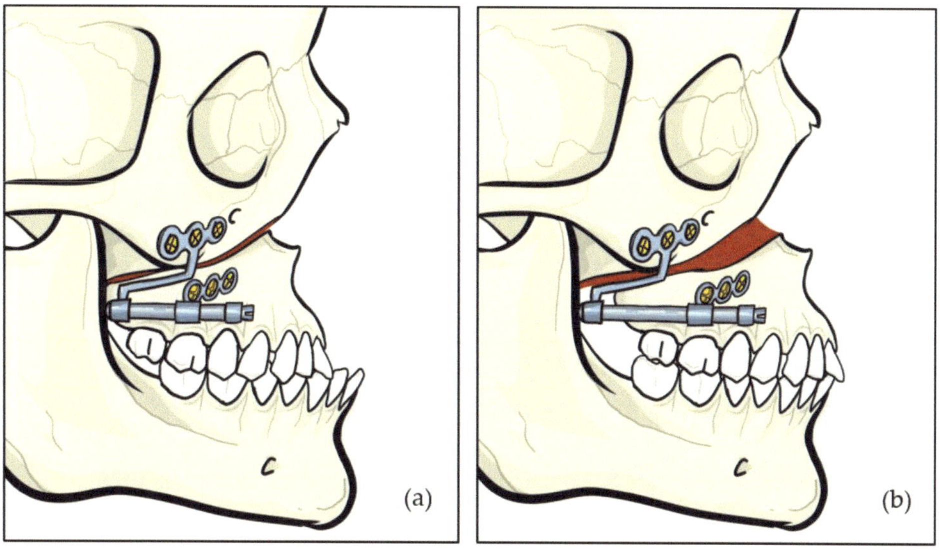

Figure 6.
Example of maxillary DO hypoplastic maxilla. (a) Application of internal distractor device following osteotomy. (b) Distracted maxilla in AP direction.

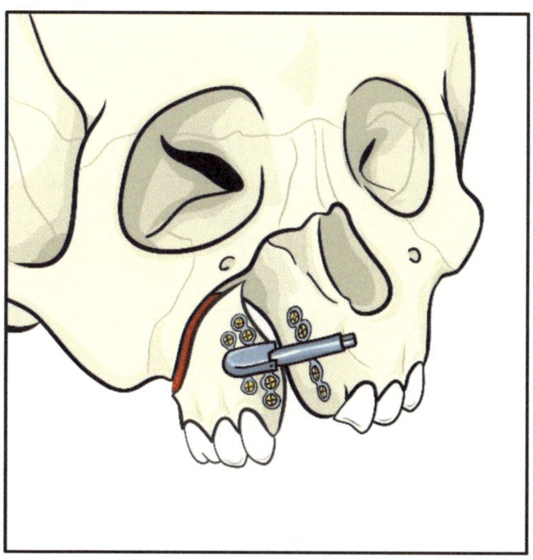

Figure 7.
Application of transport DO to reconstruct a defect in the right maxillary bone.

4.5 Craniofacial DO

Complex congenital craniofacial cases such as syndromic craniosynostosis may cause serious functional impairment (**Figure 8**). These conditions include Crouzon, Apert and Pfeiffer syndrome in which patients may suffer serious functional problems associated to increased ICP, severe exorbitism and OSA secondary to structural growth abnormality related to the early fusion of cranial sutures.

Patients with these problems often require massive segmental expansion of the skull and midface region to decompress the restricted intracranial space, achieving orbital protection and eyelid closure as well as opening up the nasopharyngeal space to treat the respective functional issues. Devices used for these cases may either be an external distractor device or internal devices or a combination of both [22].

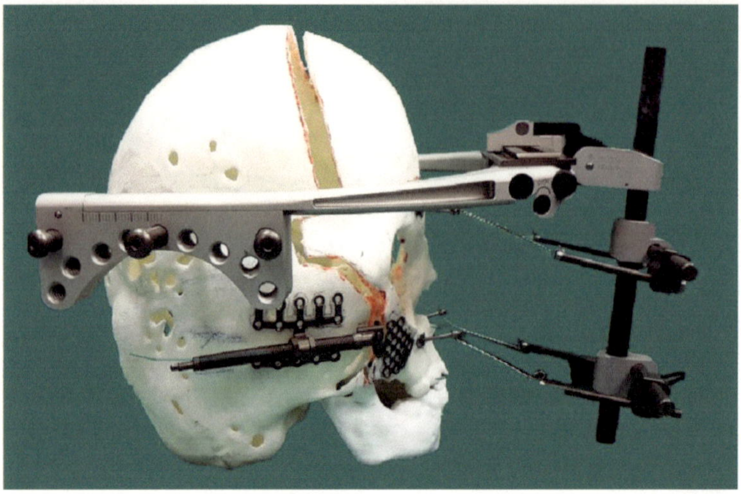

Figure 8.
Craniofacial DO in a Pfeiffer syndrome patient incorporating external and internal devices. External device in which the head frame is fixed at parietal region using percutaneous cranial pins uses pulling mechanism by wires at supraorbital and maxillary regions to advance the bone. Internal device at zygoma area uses pushing mechanism to push the bone forward. Combination of these two mechanisms provide a stable distraction of the midfacial bone with equal distribution of forces. Despite its huge size, this external device is made of lightweight aluminum, titanium and carbon fiber components for patient comfort.

5. Complications

Ever since the clinical application of DO in craniofacial region by McCarthy in 1992, this technique has been widely used to improve the morphology of the facial skeleton in patients with congenital or acquired deformities. The gradual bone distraction that leads to the regeneration of bone and simultaneous neohistogenesis eliminates the need for bone grafting procedures, thus minimizing the morbidities in the treatment of craniofacial deformities [23]. Literature cites that the complication in relation to DO is much similar to that of the other standard treatment procedures, which is up to 40% [24].

From the literature, there are numerous methods in describing complication of DO. In 1990, Paley has described problems, obstacles and complications in limb lengthening by Ilizarov technique. In 2002, Neyt et al. has adopted Paley's classification for transpalatal DO cases [25]. As for craniofacial region, Mofid et al. [26] reviewed 3278 cases and classified complications into five major categories: (1) technical failure of the distraction process, (2) injury to a vital structure, (3) failure to guide the distraction process along the appropriate vector, (4) infection and (5) 'other'.

In 2002, after reviewing 70 cases of bilateral mandibular distraction osteogenesis, van Strijen et al. [27] has divided complications into three groups: (1) intraoperative, (2) intradistraction and (3) post distraction. In 2014, Mahdah et al. [28] has adopted this classification and then further divided it into device-related and non-device related. Cheung et al. [29] has described almost similar classification in which they divided the complications into stages namely: intraoperative, latency period, active distraction and consolidation. Shetye et al. [30] reported a stratification system for mandibular osteogenesis in which incidents related to hardware or hard and soft tissue were subdivided into minor, moderate, and major.

Agarwal [31] used the same method as written by Cherkashin and Samchukov by separating the unfavorable result into error and complications. An error is an inattentive action that results in a deviation of the course of treatment thereby leading to the development of a complication whereas a complication is an unexpected deviation from the treatment plan that without appropriate correction will lead to worsening of the existing, development of a new or recurrence of the initial pathologic process. Complications of distraction can be further categorized into two categories, technical complications and specific complications.

In a systemic review paper on complications of mandibular DO, an index was developed to standardized classification that is more detailed with regards to the relevant clinical situation and possible further treatment and is more widely applicable for use by clinicians [25].

The severity and frequency of complications that may occur is correlated with the extent of the surgery. Overall, DO at craniomaxillofacial region is relatively safe. The rate of published complications in DO can vary from 27.7–40% [29]. From literature review, average percentage of complications for alveolar DO was 36.3% [32], mandibular DO ranges from 20.5% to 35.6% [33] and cumulative percentage at craniofacial region was found to be 35.6 percent [26]. Percentage of the above-mentioned complications are listed in **Table 4**.

There are few rare complications reported related to this field. Hariri et al. [23] has reported a case of eye exodeviation with limited abduction during monobloc Le Fort III DO. With regards to mandibular DO, a case of severe temporal bone resorption after mandibular DO [38] was reported and in 2017, two cases of temporomandibular joint ankylosis after early mandibular DO [39] were noted. Many of these complications can be avoided with meticulous technique and planning, but early recognition will optimize the outcomes for both patients and their family [40].

Authors (years)	Types of complications	Incidence (%)
Master et al. [33]	**Mandibular DO**	
	Relapse	64.8
	Tooth injury	22.5
	Hypertrophic scarring	15.6
	Nerve injury	11.4
	Infection	9.5
	Inappropriate distraction vector	8.8
	Device failure	7.9
	Fusion error (Premature consolidation & fibrous union)	2.4
	Temporomandibular joint injury	0.7
Mazzonetto et al. [32]	**Alveolar DO**	
	Infection	14.5
	Paresthesia	10.9
	Tipping of transport disk	5.5
	Hyperplasia	5.5
	Dehiscence	5.5
	Fracture of screw	1.8
	Fracture of device	1.8
	Osteotomy revision	1.8
	Inadequate length	1.8

Authors (years)	Types of complications	Incidence (%)
Mofid et al. [26]	**Craniofacial DO**	
	(a) *Technical failure of the distraction process*	
	Compliance	4.7
	Hardware failure	4.5
	Device dislodgement	3.0
	Premature consolidation	1.9
	Pain preventing distraction	1.0
	Fibrous union	0.5
	(b) *Damage to vital structure*	
	Inferior alveolar nerve injury	3.6
	Tooth bud injury	1.9
	Facial nerve injury	0.4
	Spinal cord injury (quadriparesis)	<0.1
	Maxillary sinus perforation	<0.1
	Parotid injury(fistula)	<0.1
	(c) *Failure to guide distraction along appropriate vector*	
	Inappropriate vector of distraction associated with single-vector distractor	8.8
	Inappropriate vector of distraction associated with single-vector distractor	7.2
	(d) *Infection*	
	Pin-tract infection or loosening	5.2
	Infection not requiring removal	2.9
	Infection requiring removal	0.9
	Osteomyelitis	0.5
	(e) *Others*	
	Chronic pain after distraction	<0.1
	Midface seroma	<0.1
Nout et al. [34]	**Rigid external distraction**	
	Frame migration (1/4 cases was traumatic migration)	28.6
	Pain at pin site	7.1
	Pin loosening	42.9
	Skin infection	7.1
	Scarring	4.8
	Decubitus of forehead	4.7
	Severe motivation problem	4.7
	Pin migration complicated with local skull fracture	4.7

Authors (years)	Types of complications	Incidence (%)
McMillan et al. [35]	**Posterior calvarial distraction**	
	CSF leaks	14
	Bleeding	2
	Incomplete osteotomies and gull winging	6
	Infection	18
	Minor wound breakdown	4
	Mechanical problem	12
	Serious complications	
	Torcula hemorrhage	2
	Cerebritis	2
	Dural tear	2
Dunaway et al. [36]	**Frontofacial distraction**	
	Mortality	<1
	Significant blood loss (greater than 1 blood volume)	5.3–9.1
	CSF leak	2–20
	Frontal bone necrosis	3–20
	CSF fistula	6.2
	Seizure	6.2
	Major blood loss	6.2
	Zygomatic fracture	6.2
von Bremen et al. [37]	**Mandibular midline distraction**	
	Instable screw	4
	Re-osteotomy	3
	Scar stricture	2
	Tooth fracture	2
	Mandibular swelling	1
	Abscess	1
	Recession	1

Table 4.
Percentage of complications in craniomaxillofacial DO.

6. Research and advances

Distraction osteogenesis offers many advantages in craniofacial surgical practice, such as the ability of correction of the deformity without the need for a bone graft [26]. Because of the advances in surgical technique and technical equipment, the indications of the DO have significantly widened [41].

There has been an explosion of distractor designs available on the market in the last 20 years. Further development is limited by the intermittent mode of distraction activation and the mechanical age may soon be replaced by biological modulation of distraction for compromised tissues and hosts. Emerging results of distraction from some new research directions are further elaborated below [29].

6.1 Automated continuous DO

Currently available distraction devices are patient and surgeon dependent. The patient must adjust the manual control two or more times daily, often over long periods. Because non-compliance and device failure are the leading causes of treatment failure, the patient requires numerous clinical visits to ensure proper distractor activation [42]. Considering these drawbacks, many research groups are working to design novel distraction devices that expand automatically and continuously. An automated mechanism would eliminate the need for patient compliance and decrease the frequency of post-operative visits for patient supervision. At the moment, the types of these devices are classified into three categories based on the method of power: hydraulic, motor-driven and spring-mediated [43–47]. It has also been reported that continuous distraction may be carried out at rates up to 2 mm per day with formation of bone in the gap. This would allow greater distraction distances in a shorter period, without sacrificing bone quality [43].

6.2 Administration of growth factors to enhance bone healing

The major disadvantage of DO is the long distraction and consolidation period, which contributes to the risk of complications such as local infection (**Figure 9**) which may jeopardize the effectiveness of DO application clinically. The major objectives in current DO research focus on the acceleration of new bone formation and shortening the treatment period. Great efforts have been made by researchers and clinicians to promote bone formation via local and systematic administration of angiogenic and osteogenic growth factors or cytokines, including bone morphogenic protein (BMP), transforming growth factor beta (TGF-β), platelet-derived growth factor (PDGF), vascular endothelial growth factor (VEGF), and fibroblast growth factor (FGF). Among all these growth factors and cytokines, BMPs play the most important role in bone healing and regeneration by inducing the osteogenic differentiation of mesenchymal stem cells and have a synergistic effect with the angiogenic growth factor, VEGF [29]. On a rabbit model of mandibular lengthening, recombinant human (rh) BMP-2 has been demonstrated to enhance bone ossification at both routine and

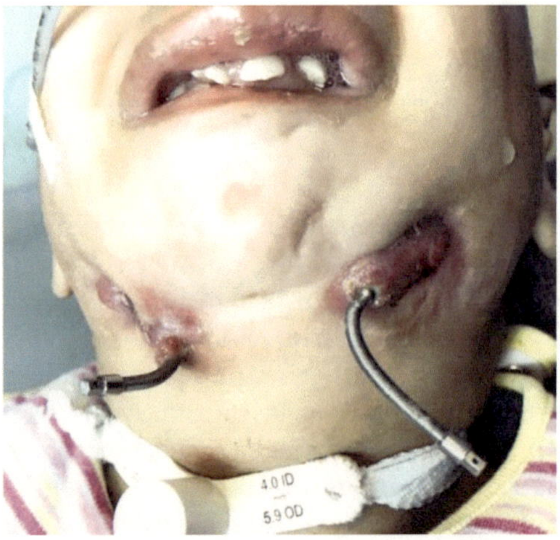

Figure 9.
Common complication of a localized infection at the exit wound of mandibular distractor's activation rods.

rapid distraction rates. The addition of rhBMP-2 was able to compensate for the rapid distraction rate in DO [46]. Nevertheless, the effectiveness of delivery method, cost and biological safety still require further investigation [29].

6.3 Development in distraction devices

In a case of complex mandibular deformities, a complex multivector extraoral device with multiple joints is used in order to achieve movements in all desired plane. This device may be difficult for the patient and surgeon to manage and errors often occur during active distraction. The use of a semi-buried curvilinear distraction device (Synthes CMF, West Chester, PA), with 3-dimensional treatment planning, is a potentially powerful tool to correct complex mandibular deformities [48].

In conclusion, DO is a reliable technique to regenerate new bone and can be considered as an effective alternative in oral and craniomaxillofacial reconstructive surgery. The technique application requires comprehensive understanding of its principles, appropriate pre-surgical planning, expert technical handling, reasonably good surgical skills, and a holistic post-surgical care in preventing potential complications.

Author details

Firdaus Hariri*, Siok Yoong Chin, Jonathan Rengarajoo, Qi Chao Foo,
Siti Nur Nabihah Zainul Abidin and Ahmad Fadhli Ahmad Badruddin
Department of Oral and Maxillofacial Clinical Sciences, Faculty of Dentistry,
University of Malaya, Kuala Lumpur, Malaysia

*Address all correspondence to: firdaushariri@um.edu.my

References

[1] Hegab AF, Shuman MA. Distraction Osteogenesis of the Maxillofacial Skeleton: Biomechanics and Clinical Implications. Vol. 1. 2012. p. 509

[2] Angell E. Treatment of irregularity of the permanent or adult teeth. Dental Cosmos. 1860;**1**:540-544, 99-600

[3] Ilizarov GA. The tension-stress effect on the genesis and growth of tissues. Part I. The influence of stability of fixation and soft-tissue preservation. Clinical Orthopaedics and Related Research. 1989;**238**:249-281

[4] Ilizarov GA. The tension-stress effect on the genesis and growth of tissues: Part II. The influence of the rate and frequency of distraction. Clinical Orthopaedics and Related Research. 1989;**239**:263-285

[5] McCarthy JG, Stelnicki EJ, Mehrara BJ, Longaker MT. Distraction osteogenesis of the craniofacial skeleton. Plastic and Reconstructive Surgery. 2001;**107**:1812-1827

[6] Swennen G, Schliephake H, Dempf R, Schierle H, Malevez C. Craniofacial distraction osteogenesis: A review of the literature. Part 1: Clinical studies. Journal of Oral and Maxillofacial Surgery. 2001;**30**:89-103

[7] Carls FR, Sailer HF. Seven years clinical experience with mandibular distraction in children. Journal of Cranio-Maxillofacial Surgery. 1998;**26**:197-208

[8] Andrade N, Gandhewar T, Kalra R. Development and evolution of distraction devices: Use of indigenous appliances for distraction osteogenesis-an overview. Annals of Maxillofacial Surgery. 2011;**1**:58-65

[9] Chin M, Toth BA. Distraction osteogenesis in maxillofacial surgery using internal devices: Review of five cases. Journal of Oral and Maxillofacial Surgery. 1996;**54**:45-53

[10] Nada RM, Sugar AW, Wijdeveld MG, Borstlap WA, Clauser L, Hoffmeister B, et al. Current practice of distraction osteogenesis for craniofacial anomalies in Europe: A web based survey. Journal of Cranio-Maxillofacial Surgery. 2010;**38**:83-89

[11] Al Ruhaimi KA. Comparison of different distraction rates in the mandible: An experimental investigation. International Journal of Oral and Maxillofacial Surgery. 2001;**30**:220-227

[12] Lin SJ, Roy S, Patel PK. Distraction osteogenesis in the pediatric population. Otolaryngology-Head and Neck Surgery. 2007;**137**:233-238

[13] Higuera S, Cole P, Stephenson JB, Hollier L. Distraction rate and latency: Factors in the outcome of paediatric maxillary distraction. Journal of Plastic, Reconstructive & Aesthetic Surgery. 2009;**62**:1564-1567

[14] Breik O, Tivey D, Umapathysivam K, Anderson P. Does the rate of distraction or type of distractor affect the outcome of mandibular distraction in children with micrognathia? Journal of Oral and Maxillofacial Surgery. 2016;**74**:1441-1453

[15] Djasim UM, Wolvius EB, Van Neck JW, Van Wamel A, Weinans H, Van Der Wal KGH. Single versus triple daily activation of the distractor: No significant effects of frequency of distraction on bone regenerate quantity and architecture. Journal of Cranio-Maxillofacial Surgery. 2008;**36**:143-151

[16] Peacock ZS, Tricomi BJ, Murphy BA, Magill JC, Kaban LB, Troulis MJ. Automated continuous distraction

osteogenesis may allow faster distraction rates: A preliminary study. Journal of Oral and Maxillofacial Surgery. 2013;**71**:1073-1084

[17] Smith SW, Sachdeva RCL, Cope JB. Evaluation of the consolidation period during osteodistraction using computed tomography. American Journal of Orthodontics and Dentofacial Orthopedics. 1999;**116**:254-263

[18] Yamaguchi K, Imai K, Fujimoto T, Takahashi M, Maruyama Y, Sakamoto H, et al. Cranial distraction osteogenesis for syndromic craniosynostosis: Long-term follow-up and effect on postoperative cranial growth. Journal of Plastic, Reconstructive & Aesthetic Surgery. 2014;**67**:e35-e41

[19] Alkan A, Ozer M, Bas B, Bayram M, Celebi N, Inal S, et al. Mandibular symphyseal distraction osteogenesis: Review of three techniques. International Journal of Oral and Maxillofacial Surgery. 2007;**36**:111-117

[20] Baur DA, Meyers AD. Distraction osteogenesis of the mandible. Available from: https://emedicine.medscape.com/article/844837-overview

[21] Shah AR, Meyers AD. Distraction osteogenesis of the maxilla. Available from: https://emedicine.medscape.com/article/844742-overview

[22] Hariri F, Azmi MN, Bahuri NF, Abdullah NA, Rahman ZA, Ganesan D. Crouzon syndrome: A case series of craniomaxillofacial distraction osteogenesis for functional rehabilitation. Journal of Oral and Maxillofacial Surgery. 2017;**76**:646.e1-646e12

[23] Hariri F, Cheung LK, Rahman ZA, Ramasamy SN, Ganesan D. A rare orbital complication of eye exodeviation with limited abduction during monobloc Le Fort III distraction osteogenesis. The Cleft Palate-Craniofacial Journal. 2015;**52**:489-493

[24] Balaji SM. Identifying complications in distraction osteogenesis. Annals of Maxillofacial Surgery. 2017;7:3-4

[25] Verlinden CR, van de Vijfeijken SE, Jansma EP, Becking AG, Swennen GR. Complications of mandibular distraction osteogenesis for congenital deformities: A systematic review of the literature and proposal of a new classification for complications. International Journal of Oral and Maxillofacial Surgery. 2015;**44**:37-43

[26] Mofid MM, Manson PN, Robertson BC, Tufaro AP, Elias JJ, Vander Kolk CA. Craniofacial distraction osteogenesis: A review of 3278 cases. Plastic and Reconstructive Surgery. 2001;**108**:1003-1114. discussion 115-107

[27] van Strijen PJ, Breuning KH, Becking AG, Perdijk FB, Tuinzing DB. Complications in bilateral mandibular distraction osteogenesis using internal devices. Oral Surgery, Oral Medicine, Oral Pathology, Oral Radiology, and Endodontics. 2003;**96**:392-397

[28] Mahdah S, Bariah K, Azmi MN, Saleh I, Nabil S, Hariri F. Distraction osteogenesis in the craniomaxillofacial region. Part II: Peri-operative issues, surgical procedure, complications and reliability. Malaysian Journal of Oral Maxillofacial Surgery. 2015;**13**:1-10

[29] Cheung LK, Chua HDP, Hariri F, Lo J, Ow A, Zheng LW. Chapter 48: Distraction osteogenesis. In: Andersson L, Kahnberg K-E, Pogrel MA, editors. Oral and Maxillofacial Surgery. 1st ed. West Sussex, United Kingdom: Wiley-Blackwell; 2010. pp. 1027-1059

[30] Shetye PR, Warren SM, Brown D, Garfinkle JS, Grayson BH, McCarthy JG. Documentation of the incidents associated with mandibular distraction:

Introduction of a new stratification system. Plastic and Reconstructive Surgery. 2009;**123**:627-634

[31] Agarwal R. Unfavourable results with distraction in craniofacial skeleton. Indian Journal of Plastic Surgery. 2013;**46**:194-203

[32] Mazzonetto R, Allais M, Maurette PE, Moreira RW. A retrospective study of the potential complications during alveolar distraction osteogenesis in 55 patients. International Journal of Oral and Maxillofacial Surgery. 2007;**36**:6-10

[33] Master DL, Hanson PR, Gosain AK. Complications of mandibular distraction osteogenesis. The Journal of Craniofacial Surgery. 2010;**21**:1565-1570

[34] Nout E, Wolvius EB, van Adrichem LN, Ongkosuwito EM, van der Wal KG. Complications in maxillary distraction using the RED II device: A retrospective analysis of 21 patients. International Journal of Oral and Maxillofacial Surgery. 2006;**35**:897-902

[35] McMillan K, Lloyd M, Evans M, White N, Nishikawa H, Rodrigues D, et al. Experiences in performing posterior calvarial distraction. The Journal of Craniofacial Surgery. 2017;**28**:664-669

[36] Dunaway DJ, Britto JA, Abela C, Evans RD, Jeelani NU. Complications of frontofacial advancement. Child's Nervous System. 2012;**28**:1571-1576

[37] von Bremen J, Schäfer D, Kater W, Ruf S. Complications during mandibular midline distraction. The Angle Orthodontist. 2008;**78**:20-24

[38] Feng S, Zhang Z, Shi L, Tang X, Liu W, Yin L, et al. Temporal bone resorption: An uncommon complication after mandibular distraction. The Journal of Craniofacial Surgery. 2015;**26**:e185-e187

[39] Galie M, Candotto V, Elia G, Clauser LC. Temporomandibular joint ankylosis after early mandibular distraction osteogenesis: A new syndrome? The Journal of Craniofacial Surgery. 2017;**28**:1185-1190

[40] Winters R, Tatum SA. Craniofacial distraction osteogenesis. Facial Plastic Surgery Clinics of North America. 2014;**22**:653-664

[41] Norholt SE, Jensen J, Schou S, Pedersen TK. Complications after mandibular distraction osteogenesis: A retrospective study of 131 patients. Oral Surgery, Oral Medicine, Oral Pathology, Oral Radiology, and Endodontics. 2011;**111**:420-427

[42] Goldwaser BR, Papadaki ME, Kaban LB, Troulis MJ. Automated continuous mandibular distraction osteogenesis: Review of the literature. Journal of Oral and Maxillofacial Surgery. 2012;**70**:407-416

[43] Kessler P, Neukam FW, Wiltfang J. Effects of distraction forces and frequency of distraction on bony regeneration. The British Journal of Oral & Maxillofacial Surgery. 2005;**43**:392-398

[44] Schmelzeisen R, Neumann G, von der Fecht R. Distraction osteogenesis in the mandible with a motor-driven plate: A preliminary animal study. The British Journal of Oral & Maxillofacial Surgery. 1996;**34**:375-378

[45] Mofid MM, Inoue N, Tufaro AP, Vander Kolk CA, Manson PN. Spring-mediated mandibular distraction osteogenesis. The Journal of Craniofacial Surgery. 2003;**14**:756-762

[46] Zheng LW, Cheung LK, Ma L, Wong MC. High-rhythm automatic driver for bone traction: An experimental

study in rabbits. International Journal of Oral and Maxillofacial Surgery. 2008;**37**:736-740

[47] Ayoub AF, Richardson W, Barbenel JC. Mandibular elongation by automatic distraction osteogenesis: The first application in humans. The British Journal of Oral & Maxillofacial Surgery. 2005;**43**:324-328

[48] Kaban LB, Seldin EB, Kikinis R, Yeshwant K, Padwa BL, Troulis MJ. Clinical application of curvilinear distraction osteogenesis for correction of mandibular deformities. Journal of Oral and Maxillofacial Surgery. 2009;**67**:996-1008